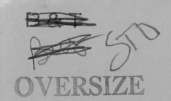

NANCY STRONG'S

AEROBIC SLIMNASTICS

NANCY STRONG'S

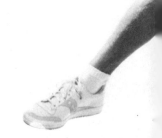

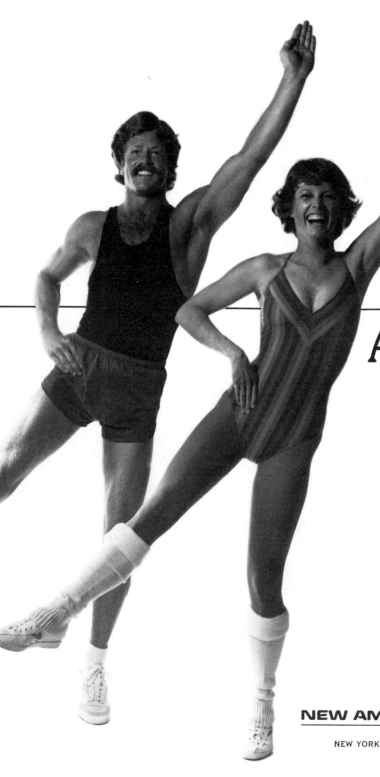

NANCY STRONG
with SUSAN HAAS LENCI
Photographs by NANCY WAYMAN

AEROBIC SLIMNASTICS

NAL BOOKS
NEW AMERICAN LIBRARY
TIMES MIRROR
NEW YORK AND SCARBOROUGH, ONTARIO

NAL BOOKS TRADEMARK REG. U.S. PAT. OFF.
AND FOREIGN COUNTRIES
REGISTERED TRADEMARK—MARCA REGISTRADA
HECHO EN HARRISONBURG, VA., U.S.A.

SIGNET, SIGNET CLASSIC, MENTOR, PLUME, MERIDIAN and NAL BOOKS are published *in the United States* by The New American Library, Inc., 1633 Broadway, New York, New York 10019, *in Canada* by The New American Library of Canada Limited, 81 Mack Avenue, Scarborough, Ontario M1L 1M8

Library of Congress Cataloging in Publication Data

Strong, Nancy.
    Nancy Strong's Aerobic slimnastics.
    Bibliography: p.
    1. Aerobic dancing.
2. Reducing exercises.
3. Reducing diets.
I. Lenci, Susan Haas.
II. Wayman, Nancy.   III. Title.
IV. Title: Aerobic slimnastics.
V. Title: Slimnastics.
RA781.15.S77 1983   613.7'1   83-11370
ISBN 0-453-00446-6

Designed by Barbara Huntley

First Printing, November, 1983

1 2 3 4 5 6 7 8 8

PRINTED IN THE UNITED STATES OF AMERICA

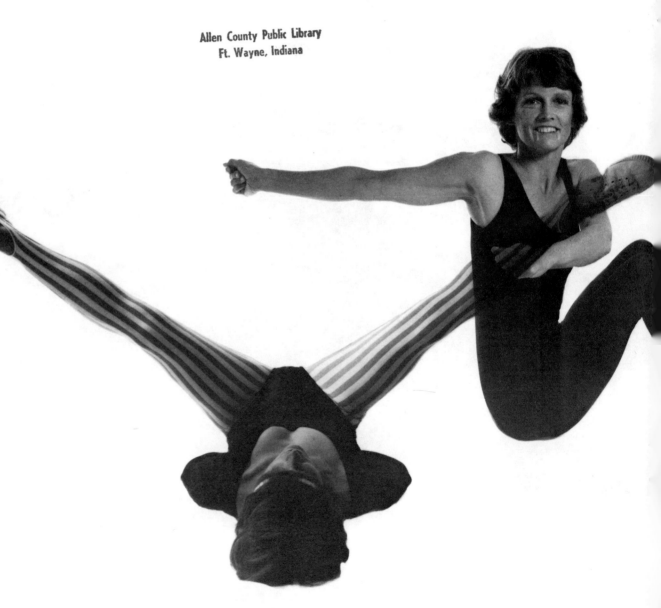

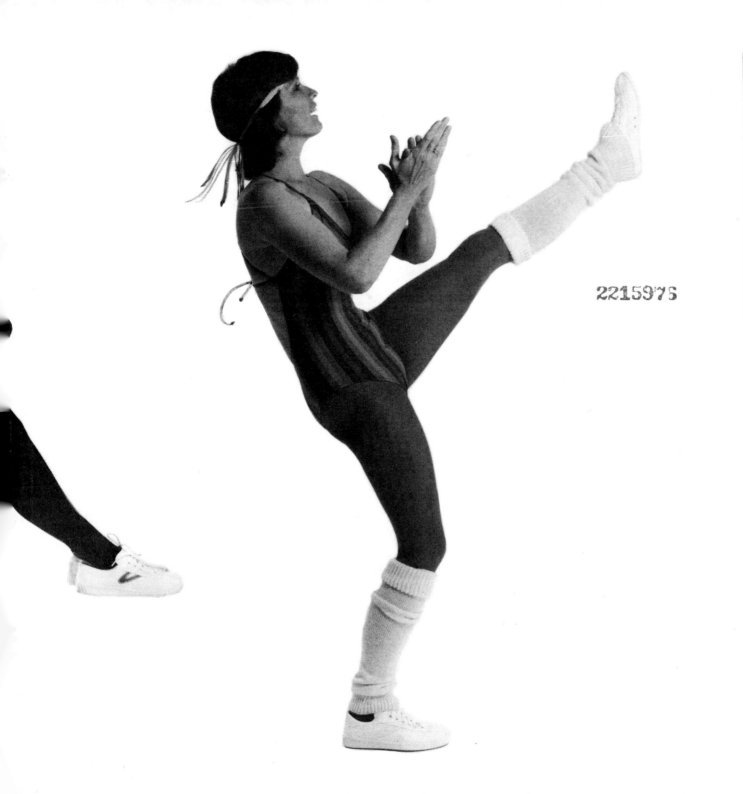

To my family—
*BRIAN, ROBBIE,
KEVIN, and DANA*—
*for their loving patience,
and to the*
FIRST FOOTERS
*for their loyal dedication
and boundless energy*

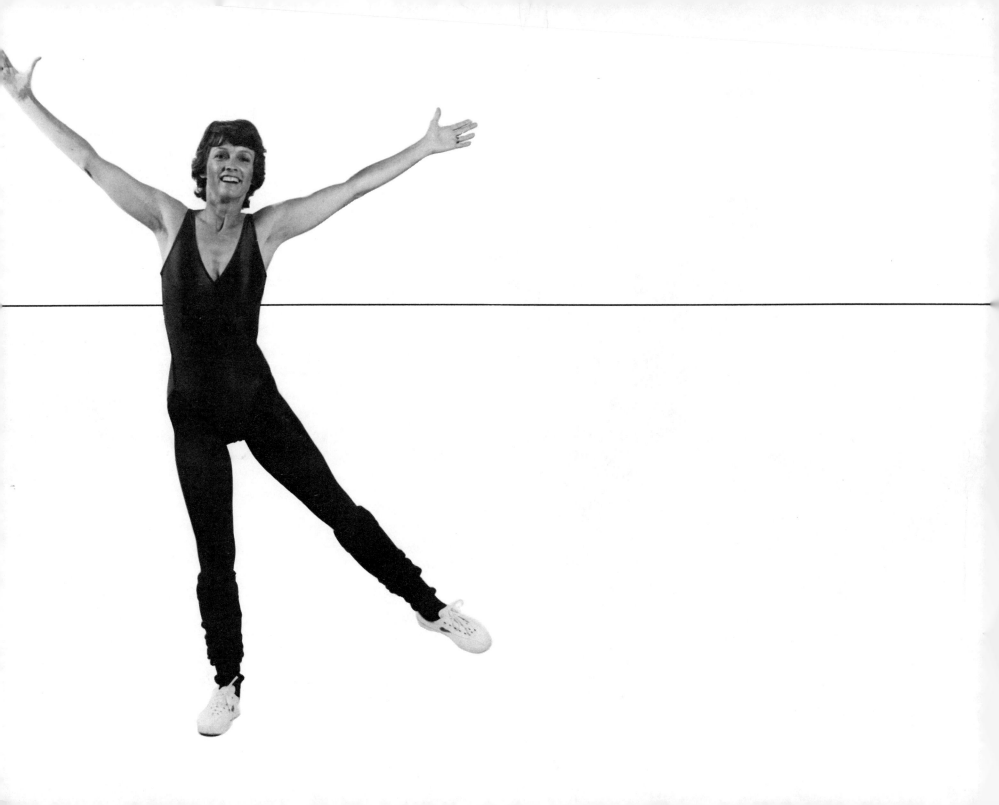

Contents

Acknowledgments

My special thanks go to all the people who made this book possible, especially the following:

Susan Haas Lenci, our writer and a full-time journalist. (Used to jogging and gymnastics, she says Aerobic Slimnastics gives her the energy to keep her busy life together.)

Nancy Wayman, our photographer. (A professional who switches between long hours standing in the darkroom and short periods of concentrated dashing around during photographic sessions, Nancy says Aerobic Slimnastics has really boosted her vitality and endurance, and "saved her life.")

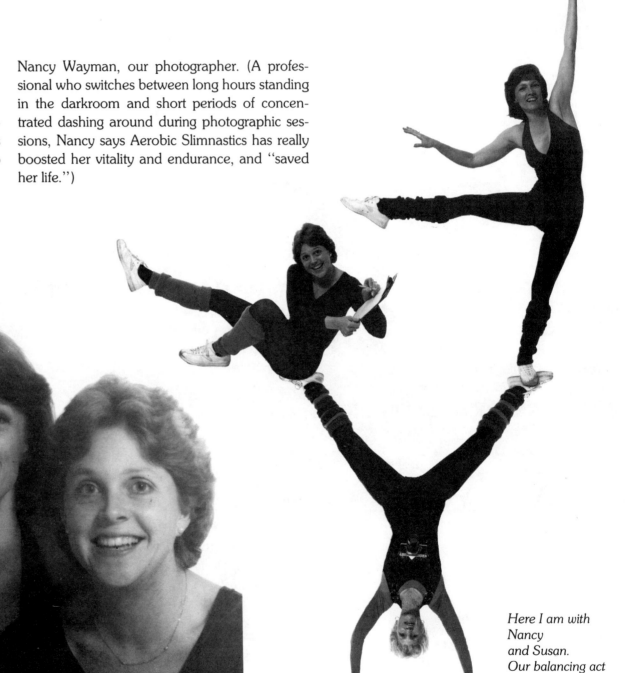

Here I am with Nancy and Susan. Our balancing act brought you this book.

The Aerobic Slimnastics office staff, who typed and retyped, cut and pasted, and stayed in great spirits with Aerobic Slimnastics workouts.

Also . . .
Myron Miller, Aerobic Slimnastics cartoonist, for his illustrations; Lucy Massey, R.D., and Kay Staid, for their nutritional expertise; Howard I. Shapiro, M.D., for his medical input; Frank Ca-

pone of Karen & Frank's House of Beauty, Westport, Connecticut, for my exercise-convenient hairstyle; and Ann Kelly and Vicki Kovel, for helping with the care of my children, pets, and home.

And . . .
All of the Aerobic Slimnastics instructors and students.

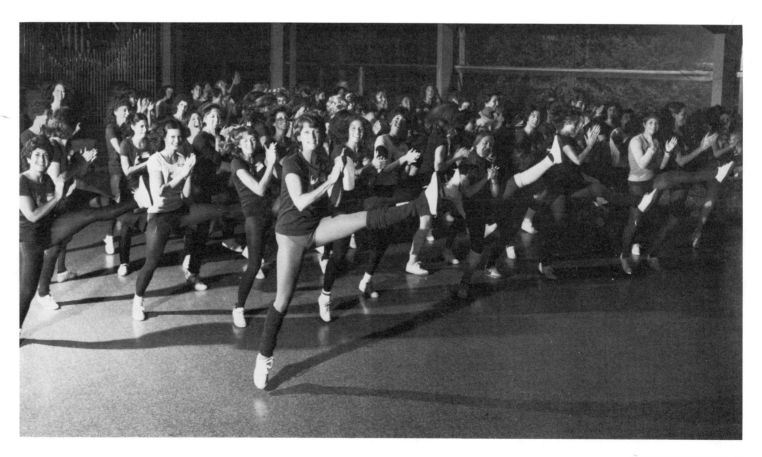

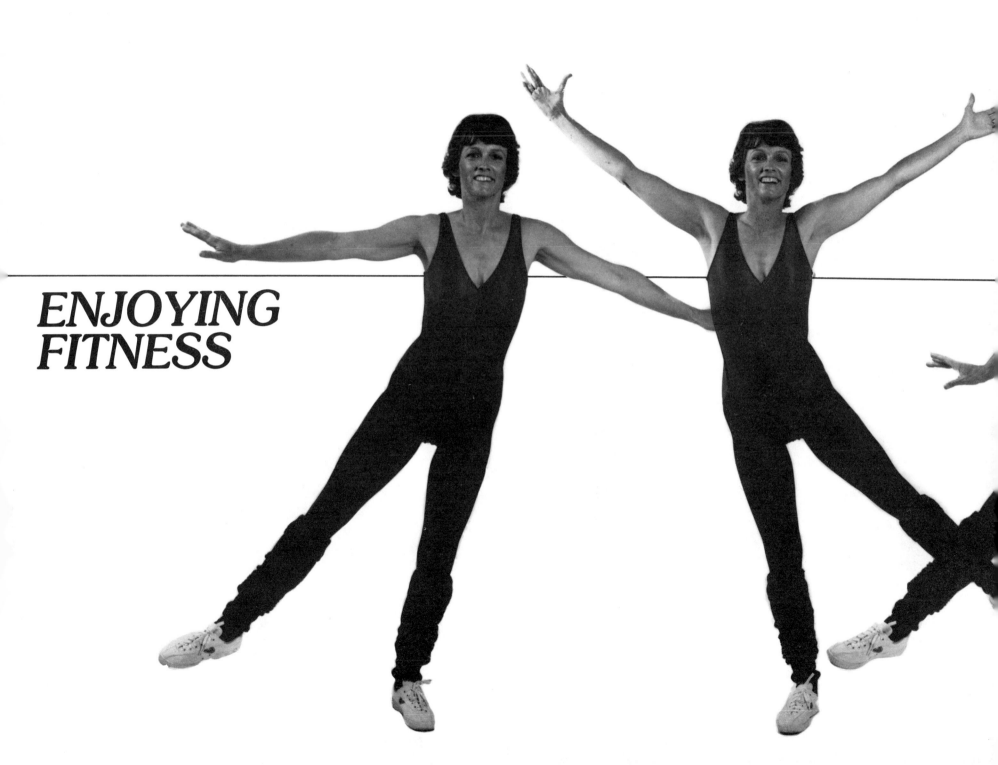

ENJOYING
FITNESS

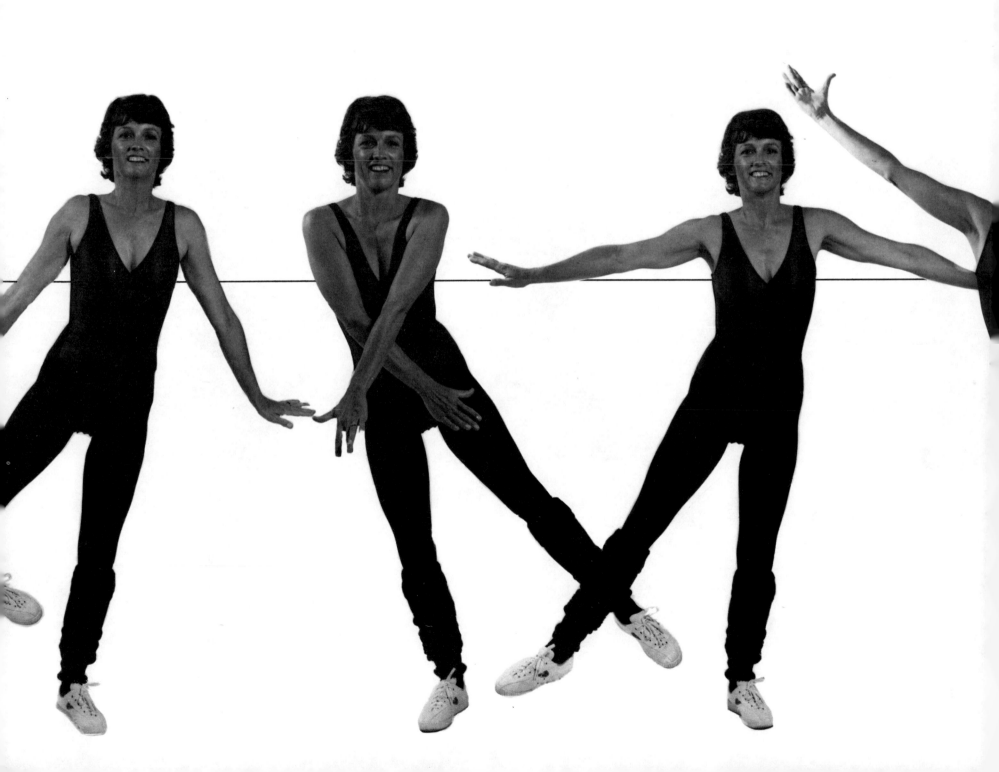

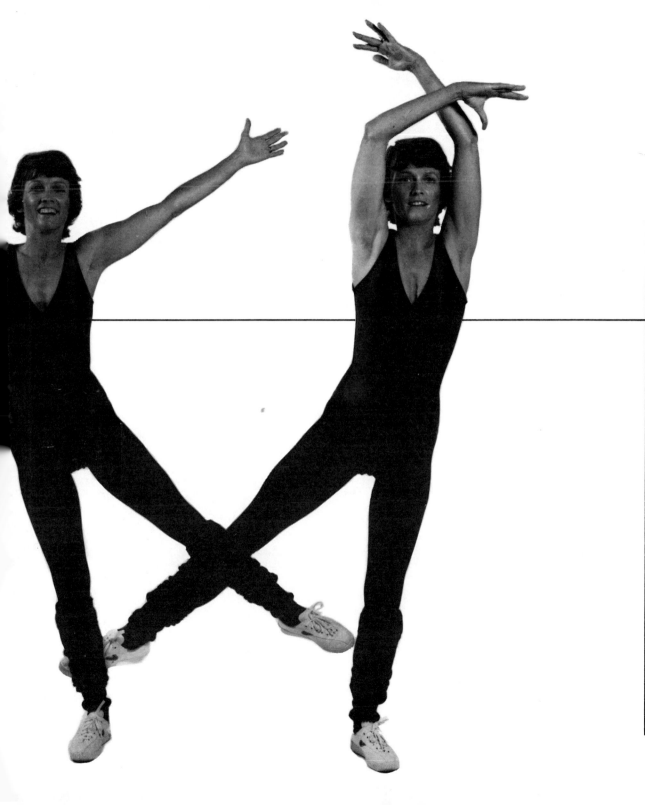

A New Way of Living

You are going to love Aerobic Slimnastics. When I close my eyes, I can picture you exercising with me and both of us feeling good. Aerobic Slimnastics brings immediate gratification. Just as soon as we finish the last exercise, you are going to feel totally energized and revitalized. I can see you walking with a spring in your step, feeling comfortable, competent, and strong. And I can picture even greater rewards for you when you make Aerobic Slimnastics a part of your life.

You are going to live your leisure time in greater depth. You are going to sleep better and awake feeling ready to tackle your day's work. You will have more energy for your children, your spouse, and your friends, and all the activities you enjoy.

Do you participate regularly in a sport? Aerobic Slimnastics will give you a total body workout and improve your stamina. I'm going to show you some exercises that will help prevent back fatigue, muscle stiffness, and knee problems. You will increase your flexibility and be more injury-resistant. Because you'll be in better shape, you'll play a better game and have more fun.

You are going to see wonderful changes in your body. You are going to slim, trim, firm, and find muscles you didn't know you had. It will be so pleasant to stand in front of your mirror and see the beautiful body you want to see. You will also seek out a healthier diet. It will be a natural outgrowth of the exercise. The section on Food Fitness will provide you with skills to design a nutritious diet that can become a lifetime eating plan. You are going to start burning more calories. So, if you are overweight, the weight you lose will stay off.

How long has it been since you exercised regularly? After today, that doesn't matter. With Aerobic Slimnastics I will help you exercise at your own pace, to start where you are now, set your own goals, and get where you want to be.

When I designed Aerobic Slimnastics I wanted to make a program that would inspire people to come to class and to make physical fitness a part of their lives. That's the way I feel about this book. It will not gather dust on your coffee table. Make it your class. This is a book you will be able to use, a program you will be able to do. Aerobic Slimnastics is simple and fun and you will feel rejuvenated. I'm not going to keep any secrets from you. I want you to know about fitness and why Aerobic Slimnastics will work for you. Aerobic Slimnastics is more than a workout. It is a way of life that will bring out the best in you. You have made your commitment. Now it's my job to motivate you to stay with the program. Join me and let's do Aerobic Slimnastics together. I'll be your instructor and I'll take good care of you.

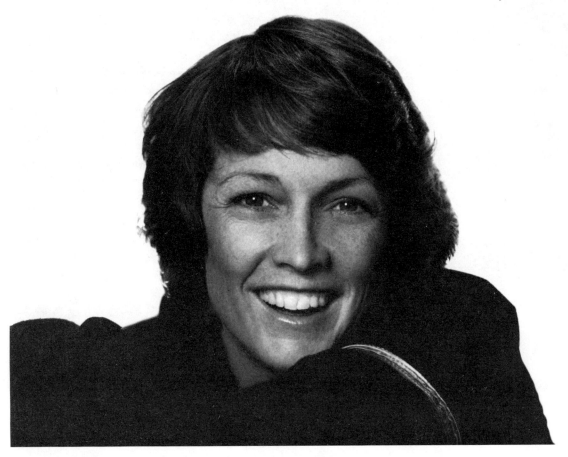

Join me and we'll do Aerobic Slimnastics together. I'll be your instructor and I'll take good care of you.

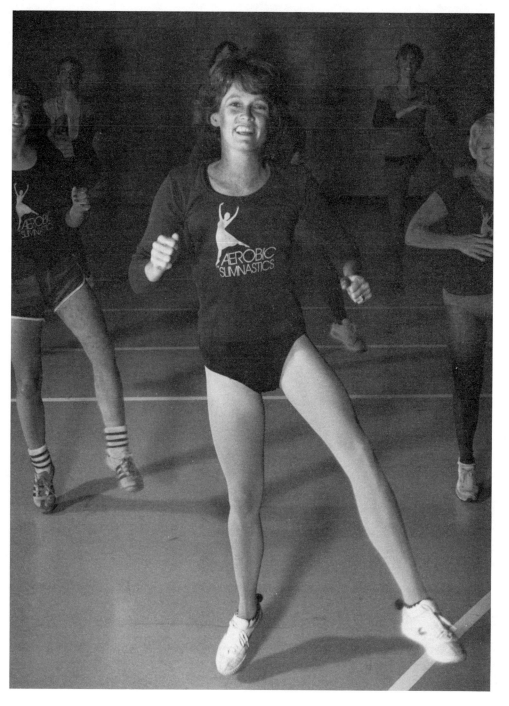

I want to confide in you about the experiences that led me to design Aerobic Slimnastics and about my overwhelming desire to make a safe and challenging fitness program that people would love.

I get such joy out of watching Aerobic Slimnastics students become strong and self-confident. As a child, I was very active but I was not athletic. I had very little training—no tennis lessons, no swimming lessons, not even the informal structure of a neighborhood baseball team. In my family, we never discussed the importance of exercise. I had about a year of ballet lessons, but the idea behind them was to make a lady out of me, not to make me fit or strong. That was the extent of it. When I became an adult and looked around for a way to keep fit, I had no background. I couldn't play racquet sports or golf and was not a good enough swimmer to do laps. I was trying to find a fitness program for me, but flopping around from one thing to another— swimming, ballet, yoga. I couldn't do anything well enough to be comfortable and stick with it.

Whatever class I was involved in, I always felt extremely uncoordinated and self-conscious. I finally took a jazz dance class in a small local shopping center school in Florida where we were living. I was the only adult enrolled. I danced with the children. The director made such a fuss over me—the one "mommy." There I was with the children, who danced so effortlessly. I stuck out like a sore thumb. Where was everybody my age? In the 1960s, there was a lot of talk about politics, pot and protest, but little about physical fitness. Active people were trying to get in shape with sports, but few considered shaping up before playing. In sparsely attended exercise classes, the emphasis for most women was on developing a nice figure for someone else to look at rather than exercising to become strong and fit.

My first pregnancy with our son Robbie changed my life in more ways than one. Desiring to be awake and aware and in control at his birth, I enrolled in a Lamaze prepared-childbirth class. The teachers were convinced that the right kind of exercise could make a difference for a woman and her body. I was so excited to be with people who thought that way. I was learning to exercise so I could take charge and do something for myself, and that was the first time I had ever come across that philosophy so clearly stated.

There was little time to follow through on my new insight, as our second child, Kevin, was born one year later. It was about this time that people began to talk a little about jogging. You didn't see many people running on the streets, but some people were talking and writing about this new sport, and I began doing some of my own research into exercise physiology. I also put on my sneakers and tried to run a half-mile around the block. I couldn't do it. I fantasized that a mugger was chasing me and I had to run for my life. I was twenty-eight years old and couldn't make my legs move. This experience, terrifying and frustrating, convinced me to start looking again for an exercise program.

When a local Y offered a slimnastics class with baby-sitting, I arrived, babies in tow, ready to shape up a new me. You can imagine how disappointed I was when the director announced the teacher had resigned. There stood twelve mommies, assorted babies, and the baby-sitter. Panicked, I said, "Don't dismiss the baby-sitter!

I'll teach the class." My career was launched! With the general pattern of Aerobic Slimnastics already in mind, I structured the class with a warm-up, some exercises to get us out of breath, and slimnastics to tone hips, thighs, and tummies. In my experience with other exercise classes, the teachers weren't doing the job. They were not selling fitness. The students were there, but they didn't love it. The missionary zeal that I had experienced with my Lamaze teachers, the belief that exercise could make a real difference in the lives of students, wasn't evident in most exercise classes. I wanted to design a safe and challenging class that students would love so that they would want to come back.

After the birth of our daughter, Dana, we moved to Georgia to a contemporary house in the woods. We had no money for furniture, so the large first floor was impossible to live in, but it made a great exercise studio. Before long, I had thirty students and a play group for the babies in Dana's room. Leaving for work, my husband, Brian, would often encounter leotard-clad ladies in his living room, dining room, and kitchen!

Next stop—Tokyo. A two-year assignment in Japan with Brian's company gave me the opportunity to try my program on an international mix of women at the Tokyo American Club. The universal appeal of exercise allowed me to experience different cultures, many of which encouraged women to exercise not just to be thin and gorgeous but to be strong and healthy. For the Japanese, fitness is a nationalistic happening. They are not exercising to trim figures, but to build healthy minds, bodies, and spirits, and, as a result, a healthy nation. All around me, the Japanese were biking, hiking, jogging, skiing, and

doing calisthenics in parks, in schools, and in their workplaces. The culture was very supportive of my thinking, because the Japanese were so concerned with physical fitness.

When we returned to Connecticut from Tokyo, it was obvious there had been a big change in the American attitude toward fitness in the two years we were overseas. The streets were crowded with joggers. The media, fashions, and enrollment in exercise classes reflected this change in the national pastime. A sedentary nation was getting on its feet. Once the oddball in left field, I was beginning to feel in the mainstream of a national trend.

Our household was settled in Westport, Connecticut, in record time so I could jump back into teaching again. During the two years abroad I had lost touch with what American women were doing, so I began doing my own market research. I started Aerobic Slimnastics classes at all different times to test the interest. I taught four to six class hours a day. I would come home after a class, take a nap, get up, teach another class, and, in between, care for my family. I was so busy, but I was feeling wonderful—I was finding out about my market and having fun seeing how fit I could get. I felt years younger. I liked the way I looked and the way I felt. I could run fast when I wanted to, I could play with my children, and I could enjoy competitive sports with women and men. I had no more athletic skills than I had before, but my stamina was soaring for the first time in my life. At age thirty-five, I was able to do things I should have done fifteen years before! I felt self-confident and liberated, and I was catching up with the women's movement. Being physically fit, I could do anything.

Happily, as my many classes grew, I discovered that I could teach other people to teach Aerobic Slimnastics. My new instructors, whom I nicknamed the First Footers, loved their work. I was training teachers who believed as I do that people can change their lives with exercise. I found that good instructors can't be performers; they must forget about themselves and become totally aware of their students. This initial group of fitness missionaries and I were committed to building something meaningful together. Everyone felt a part of the teaching, a part of the commitment to the public, and a part of the fledgling business.

As Aerobic Slimnastics classes grew, husbands and boyfriends came to see what all the excitement was about. They expected a ladies' social hour until they put on their tennis shoes and we worked them out. Impressed, exhausted, and exhilarated, these men began to enroll in classes. I was not going to keep them out! I talked to more men who felt outside of the fitness movement because they were not involved in team sports. Many had not done anything but sit home and watch television while the rest of the country was getting fit, and they were feeling guilty. Even their wives and children were talking about running

races and exercise classes. They wanted to join in, but there was no place for them. So we made a place. We created a men's program, adjusting the exercise routines to make them feel more comfortable. Coed classes quickly became very popular because couples who worked found it very enjoyable to spend their free time exercising together.

Aerobic Slimnastics has grown into a program for everyone. We have a tots' and an elementary school program that stresses large muscle development, nutrition, and the importance of a healthy heart. Our high school program helps

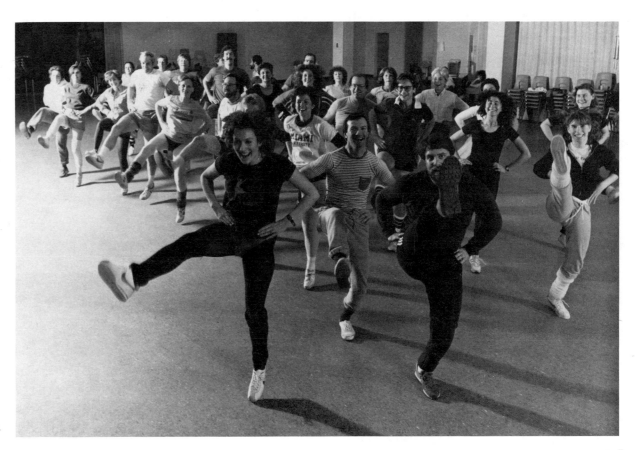

Aerobic Slimnastics is a workout for everyone.

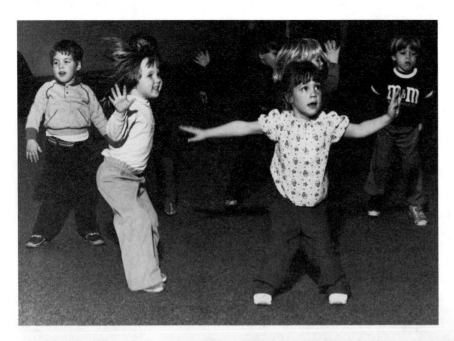

We are born with the need to exercise.

Physical fitness can last a lifetime.

teens develop cardiovascular fitness and enjoy and strengthen their rapidly changing bodies. When I was growing up, I was told to slow down and rest if I was slightly breathless. I remember my parents saying, "Be careful, you'll have a heart attack." I'd like children to understand aerobic training at a young age and to make a lifetime habit of working to strengthen their bodies.

At the other end of life, our senior citizen students are enjoying renewed energy in an Aerobic Slimnastics program modified to meet their needs. No longer do they feel obligated to fulfill the role of sedentary grandparents in rocking chairs. Exercise creates new options for them.

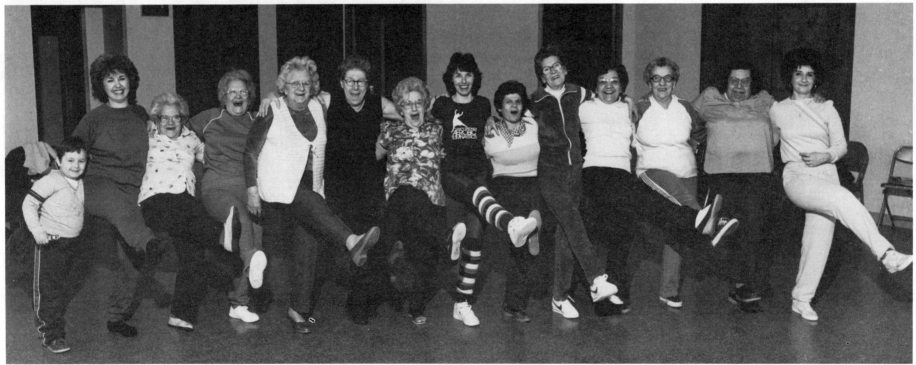

The first Aerobic Slimnastics office was a one-room arrangement in my home. The business paraphernalia spread like a creeping vine into the living room, dining room, kitchen, bedrooms, and even the bathroom. In the morning, we'd start out in one room, but gradually the staff of nine would spread their work out on the kitchen table, the dining room table, and the coffee table. Our pets—a dog, two cats, and a parrot—added to the confusion. The parrot flew over the stacks of papers, the dog announced each delivery, and the cats rode on the copier. I remember one day when I had to schedule a meeting with instructors and there wasn't one spot left in the house except upstairs on our bed. There we sat cross-legged in the middle of the bed with a portable blackboard propped up on pillows. What a way to run a business! Each day at 4:55 P.M. everyone would pack up their Aerobic Slimnastics office material and shove it under couches and beds, and by five the house would look like a home again. If someone from my family was sick or wanted to come home early, he or she certainly wasn't alone! When the children were small, it was convenient because there was always someone at home. Pity Brian, however, if he came home before five; he couldn't even park in the driveway, and, once inside, he had to step over secretaries, boxes, and projects. The fun part of all the confusion was watching a salesman come in and try to do his standard sales pitch with birds, secretaries, dogs, cats, and children all around. Many times I went so quickly from being the mother in the kitchen making peanut butter sandwiches to an executive that I was still in my bathrobe.

The business has grown up with my family. Brian has gradually become addicted to fitness.

Now he plays racquetball five or six times a week, has quit smoking, and has adjusted his diet. I'm not sure whether it was living with Aerobic Slimnastics and me that changed him or the sheer joy of fitness. We started the children in swimming lessons when they were very small, and suddenly, in the past few years, they have also become totally fitness oriented. Physical fitness is all around them and they are very serious about it. As a family, we are united in this activity. Aerobic

Slimnastics has been good for everyone. Inclined to be a "super-mom" because I am a high-energy person, I would probably have been tying shoelaces when my children were twenty-one. As a working mom, I don't have the time anymore to do and do and do for them. Now they tie their own laces, bike to their own appointments, and keep their lives in order. They are independent people, and my role as a loving parent is in better perspective.

Meet my family: my husband, Brian; our daughter, Dana; our sons, Kevin and Robbie; and our dog, Coco.

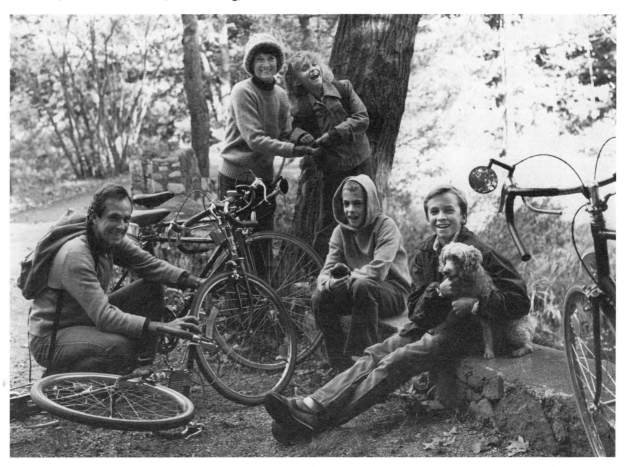

As class enrollment grew from eight original students to over thirty-thousand in three years, Aerobic Slimnastics outgrew the home office and we were forced to look for a new space. We found a seven-room office within biking distance of my home. Even in this more official setting, Aerobic Slimnastics continues to be a place for pets, children dropping in after school, and flexible work schedules. I have great confidence in the office staff and the instructors. This confidence is a key ingredient in a successful small business. The office spirit is up because everyone exercises. I'd like to invite some corporate executives into the office to show them the high morale and the work output here. And, of course, the instructors, exercising many hours a week, have boundless energy and enthusiasm.

That's the wonder of this business and the wonder of physical fitness. Everyone feels so good. For me the joy of fitness is the well-being of the instructors, staff, students, and *you!*

* * *

A typical student reaction:
"I have the vitality to accomplish in one day what used to require a week's worth of effort."

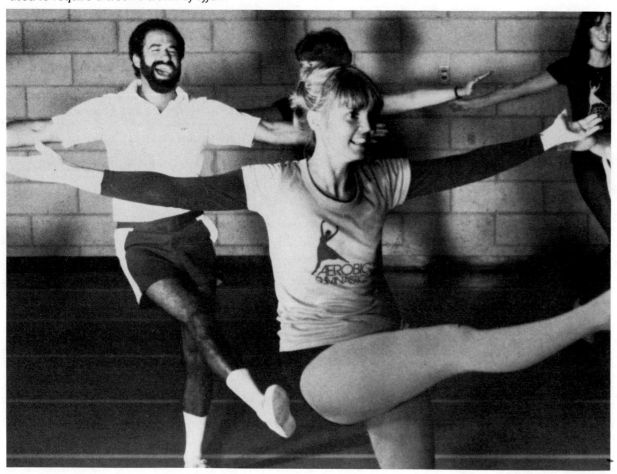

Getting Aerobic

A vigorous overall workout is aerobic if it exercises the cardiovascular system: the lungs, the muscles of the respiratory system, and the heart. The heart is the most important of the 650 muscles in your body; the one on which all others depend. A four-chambered muscle about the size of your clenched fist, the heart is a fascinating piece of body machinery, pumping blood to supply your entire circulatory system with nourishment. Like any other muscle, your heart will become stronger and more efficient with exercise.

An improved figure and spirit are not the only benefits of Aerobics Slimnastics. Another plus for aerobic training is that your heartbeat can be measured so that definite cardiovascular goals are possible. In general, a sedentary person's heart can only pump small volumes of blood with weak, short, inefficient beats. The exercised heart is much more efficient, pumping more blood with fewer, more powerful beats per minute. A person who exercises aerobically may have a resting heart rate of 20–25 beats per minute slower than a sedentary individual. Just imagine—that person conserves twelve to thirteen million beats in a year.

While strengthening your heart, aerobic exercise also helps you reduce blood pressure. It increases the flexibility and number of blood vessels. Your heart itself also develops a more complex capillary network. Apparently, aerobic exercise changes your blood chemistry by reducing the level of fats, or triglycerides, thus decreasing the tendency to form plaques that can clog blood vessels in your heart and brain.

Your cardiovascular system is a finely tuned network. Oxygen must constantly be delivered to your muscles since it cannot be stored. After the food you eat is digested and broken down, the components mix with the oxygen in your blood to produce the energy that keeps you going. During strenuous activity, your heart beats faster to supply the extra oxygen needed by your muscles. When the oxygen supply is inadequate, you will slow down until you catch your breath. Regular aerobic exercise will affect your endurance by increasing your lungs' capacity to receive more air with each breath and your heart's efficiency at pumping oxygen-filled blood. Waste products formed during exercise will slow your muscular response. Your blood, therefore, does several jobs—it delivers the oxygen and nutrients and it removes the wastes so the muscles can function smoothly. Exercising your muscles at a higher rate than you're accustomed to will tire them. But with rest, those same muscles reset themselves to a slightly higher potential. In this way, Aerobic Slimnastics, a system of exercise routines that alternates overload and rest, will take your muscles to remarkable levels of strength and endurance.

Looking Good and Feeling Better

The only way to lose fat is to burn off more calories than you take in. If you're tempted to work on your flabby thighs or tummy with a belt vibrator or roller, save your money. These gadgets are not only useless in spot reducing and weight loss but they also shake up your insides. To lose just one pound, you would have to sit through fifteen minutes of vibration every day for a year, taking Sundays off just to get rid of your headache! Spot reducing does not work. Researchers at the University of California analyzed the layer of fat in the arms of a number of regular tennis players. The right tennis arm in right-handed players had the same amount of fat as the left arm. Apparently, the extra exercise had no effect on fat in the exercised arm.

If you exercise vigorously and don't increase your calories, your body will use up fat for fuel. Be patient when you weigh yourself in the early weeks of Aerobic Slimnastics. As you begin to use fat for fuel, your body may retain some water weight. In about three weeks your body will adjust and eliminate excess fluid through urination and perspiration. Remember also that muscle weighs more than fat, so the losses may initially show up on your tape measure and not the scale.

Fat is a freeloader, putting extra demands on your heart without doing any work. Fat is also heavy to carry around and gets in your way. Cellulite is just a fancy name for fat. It develops in pockets, with fibrous bands between them, creating the perplexing cottage cheese effect. No one really knows what causes the formation of cellulite, but it may be related to poor circulation. Cellulite accumulates when the muscles are unused and the circulation is sluggish. Heredity also affects how and where you store your fat.

Muscles, on the other hand, work for us. When you exercise unused muscles, the number of blood vessels increases. The heart can then send more oxygen-filled blood to those areas needing energy for movement. The blood carries away toxins that accumulate during this metabolic process. At the same time, your muscles are toning up. Instead of sagging, these areas become firm, contributing significantly to inch loss. Amazed students say, "I haven't lost a pound, but my pants size has gone from a fourteen to a ten!" The Slimnastics part of Aerobic Slimnastics is calisthenics designed to exercise muscles that need extra toning in such problem areas as the abdominals, hips, inner thighs, and back of the upper arm. Emphasizing these muscle groups during the vigorous aerobic calorie-burning workout is the way to inch and weight loss.

Some of my students have asked if exercise will build bulky muscles. Experiments prove that vigorous athletic training for women definitely increases their strength but does not significantly change the size of the muscles. Most women do not have enough testosterone, the male hormone that affects muscle growth, to create bulky, bulging muscles. The rhythmic aerobic exercises—dancing, skipping rope, cross-country skiing, running, swimming, biking, rowing—build long muscles and a firm figure. These muscles are curvy and beautiful.

· ·

Staying Healthy with Water

I want to tell you about a surprising but key ingredient in a successful exercise program—water. Water is considered such an important part of my program that Aerobic Slimnastics instructors bring cups to class and press them into the hands of students after the workout session, continually reminding them to keep drinking! Drink six to eight eight-ounce glasses per day for good health. If this is new to you, work up to it gradually. But do it and do it with WATER.

As important as it is to your health, water is often not given the credit it deserves. It usually has no color, no smell, no flavor, and it never has any calories. Being so readily available, it's easy to take for granted. Yet water is so essential to life that it can never be eliminated, even in the most extreme fad diets. You can live quite awhile without food, depending upon the amount of body fat you have, but you can't live for more than two or three days without water.

Your body is actually two-thirds water despite its outwardly solid appearance. Each of us begins development in our mother's liquid-filled womb, and our bodies are 85 percent water at birth. Water lubricates joints and keeps body tissues soft. It also transports oxygen and other nutrients to body cells. Water is necessary for absorption and digestion of food and for the processing of waste products. Your kidneys and bladder work hard to eliminate wastes, but their job is impossible without water. Many of us know too well the aches, burning, and fever that accompany bladder and kidney infections. Thick, dark, yellow, odoriferous urine is usually a sign of insufficient water consumption and a warning that you should immediately increase your intake. Drinking water and eating fibrous food will also ease constipation, since fiber increases the stool's capacity to hold water.

THE BODY'S COOLING SYSTEM

Water protects your body against overheating. Since normal body temperature is 98.6 degrees Fahrenheit and the body becomes endangered at over 104 degrees, there is only a five-degree cushion—so your internal cooling system is extremely important. Perspiration, the positive sign of a good workout, cools the body as it evaporates. My Aerobic Slimnastics instructors are soaked after a class, dripping with perspiration. As you become more fit, your inner cooling system becomes more efficient and turns on earlier in a workout. You will also perspire at a lower body temperature, allowing you to work harder while maintaining a safe temperature. Since evaporation is responsible for the cooling process, resist the temptation to wipe the sweat from your brow on a humid day. Leave parts of the body uncovered so that perspiration can evaporate. Avoid the ''sauna suit'' that claims to ''melt away inches without exercising or dieting'' by ''sealing in your body heat''; it can create dangerous overheating. Let nature do its job.

The importance of water to you when you exercise becomes even more apparent when you consider the amount sweated off during a strenuous workout. In addition to perspiring, you lose water through the lungs as you huff and puff during a vigorous session. On hot days, marathon runners have been known to lose up to fourteen pounds of water weight, which is the reason you see them drinking at water stations during a race. If you feel tired, achy, or ''down,'' you may be dehydrated. You can test for dehydration by pulling up the skin on the back of your hand. If it springs back, your hydration is good. If it returns slowly, you may be drying out. Since we don't feel as thirsty in cold weather as we do on warm days, we frequently neglect our winter water requirements. Chapped lips are often a sign of dehydration.

You feel thirsty when salty blood, searching desperately for more water, draws water from the salivary glands and leaves the mouth dry. Brain cells receive signals from salty blood that more water is needed. When I exercise, I get a loud and clear message from my body that I am drying out; from deep inside comes an overwhelming desire for water that blocks out all other messages.

Since thirst is often quenched before the body's need for water is fulfilled, the dry mouth sensation is not always a good indicator. Merely rinsing out the mouth to satisfy thirst during exercise will not fulfill the body's need for water. The old coach's tale that drinking water during exercise will cause cramps is not necessarily so. During Aerobic Slimnastics, drink when you feel the need. If it is a very warm day and you are working hard, you should take a drink every fifteen minutes.

If you drink more than ten minutes before you begin Aerobic Slimnastics, you may find yourself with a full bladder during exercise. Take time to

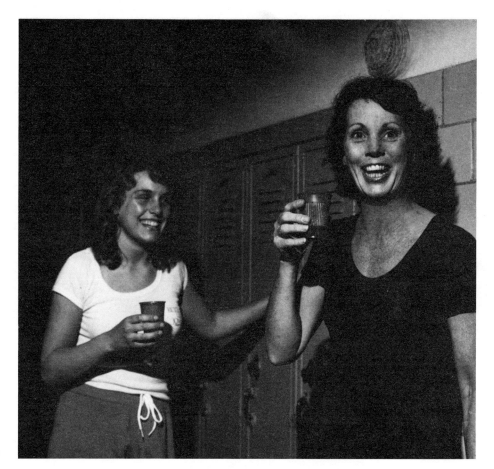

Water is a key ingredient in a successful exercise or weight-control program.

go to the bathroom. It does not build fortitude to wait; it's uncomfortable, unhealthy, and distracting. Drink one cup of water less than ten minutes before exercising to avoid the bathroom distraction. Once exercise begins, blood moves away from your kidneys to the muscles and skin, slowing urine production. Water retention problems? The good news is that you can still drink water. Retention is related to your estrogen balance and not to the amount of liquid consumed.

By now I'm sure that thirst has overcome you and you are sipping one of your daily glasses of water. Food does provide some of our daily water requirements, but I recommend an additional six to eight glasses a day. Schedule your drinks so they become part of your routine. While driving, I always take along a plastic mug of water. Do not count coffee, tea, and cola drinks as part of your six to eight glasses of water. The caffeine in these drinks is a diuretic that washes water and vital salts from your body. It also causes the blood vessels to constrict, forcing the heart to work harder at pumping blood. The headaches frequently associated with caffeine withdrawal are part of the body's reaction to the lack of constriction as the blood vessels return to normal size. Alcohol also steals vital water from the body, as anyone who has ever experienced the dry mouth of a hangover will testify. Sugar-filled drinks can cause problems for the active person since they upset blood sugar levels and dissipate important B vitamins, and the sugar that remains in the stomach can cause bloating and cramping during exercise. Sugar-free sodas are usually full of artificial coloring, flavoring, and preservatives, and can contain habit-forming caffeine. I am resistant to commercial "sport drinks"; most contain too much sugar and chemical additives and have fewer minerals than orange juice.

If everyday tap water bores you, there are positive alternatives. Inexpensive and simple seltzer is my favorite because it contains no artificial additives and is low in sodium. In addition, there is some research that suggests carbonation speeds up the stomach's absorption of fluid. Carbonation adds zip to water and provides a feeling of celebration. Look for natural spring water bottled directly from the source. Spring fresh or sparkling natural water has often had the carbonation artificially introduced. Watch the labels. Club soda, for example, is processed tap water with forced carbonation and salt additives. Try mild decaffeinated herb teas or a teaspoon of fruit juice in your water. Store a jug of water in the refrigerator. Keep these interesting variations in mind as you drink your six to eight glasses of life-sustaining water.

Now with your glass of water nearby, let's get ready for Aerobic Slimnastics.

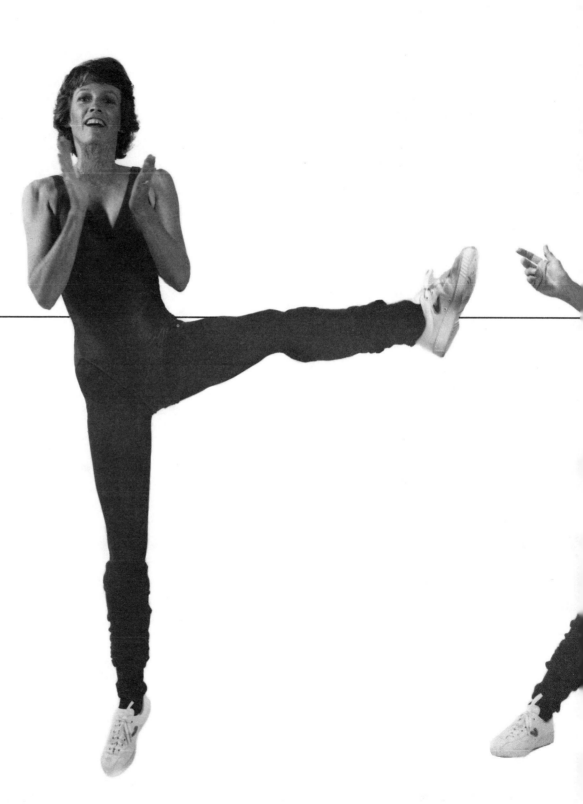

GETTING READY FOR AEROBIC SLIMNASTICS

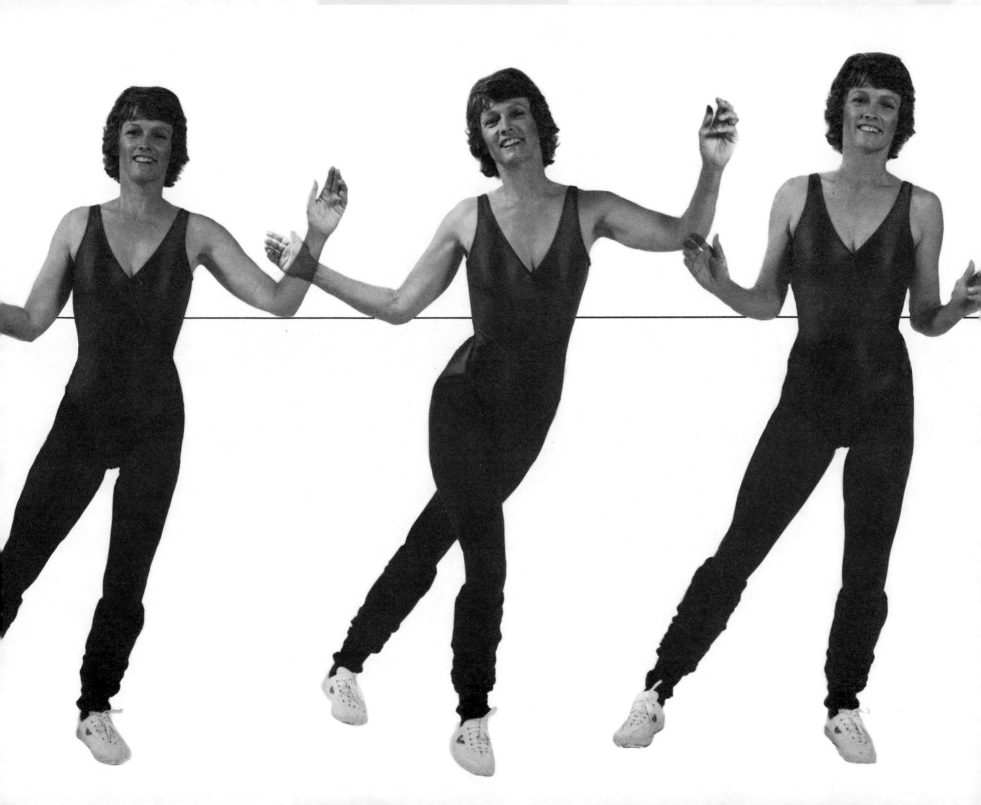

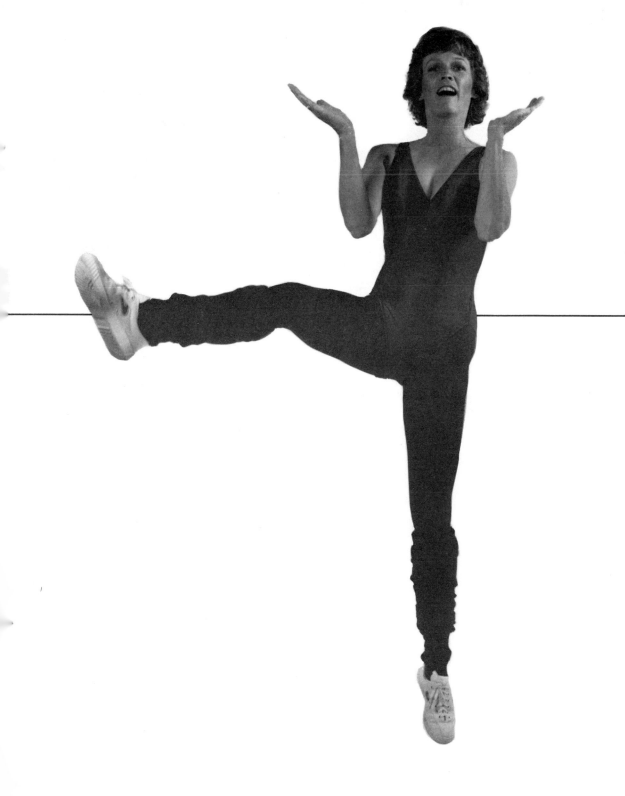

Using This Book

Once you are familiar with Aerobic Slimnastics, you'll be able to do all the routines we demonstrate in about one hour. If you are like most of my students, it will take you about eight weeks to master the entire program, but you'll start having fun and feeling better right away.

Each routine consists of exercises to be set to music of your choice. Sometimes the exercises flow together into dance patterns indicated by the dotted line that continues from page to page between music suggestions in the exercise section. Watch for the triangular arrows that indicate when the specific exercises start and the squares that show when they end, and feel free to repeat exercises several times if you like before continuing with the routine. Large squares indicate when routines end. The routines are arranged in a sequence that will give you the maximum conditioning benefit.

WARMING UP FOR THE BIG TIME

Starting with a gentle, rhythmic, total-body warm-up, you'll move on to a brisk walk that allows you to practice exercises that will be repeated later at a more aerobic pace. After stretching your legs at a chair, barre, or wall, and warming up your pelvic, abdominal, and lower back muscles, you'll be ready to *go*.

LET'S DANCE

Doing the Disco picks up the beat aerobically. Your heart and lungs will begin to work harder as you dance through the exercises.

THE BIG TIME!

With these aerobic workouts you will learn to monitor your pulse, and working at your own level, you'll condition your heart and lungs.

FANTASTIC SLIMNASTICS

Stimulating exercises will *zero in* on the challenging areas, toning and firming your upper arms, waist, hips, buttocks, abdominals, and thighs.

GOOD HEALTH AND GOOD SEX

Exercise your pelvic, abdominal, and lower back muscles—the muscles that hold you up *inside* and *out*. Strengthened, these muscles can make living more comfortable and sex more enjoyable.

Now I'd like you to meet the people who will help me show you how to do Aerobic Slimnastics. Think of us in front of you, as if we were your mirror images. When the written instructions say "Raise your right arm," for instance, you will see one of us facing you raising a left arm in the photograph. Of course, if our backs are to you or we are facing sideways, we'll be pictured working the same side that you are told to work in the written directions.

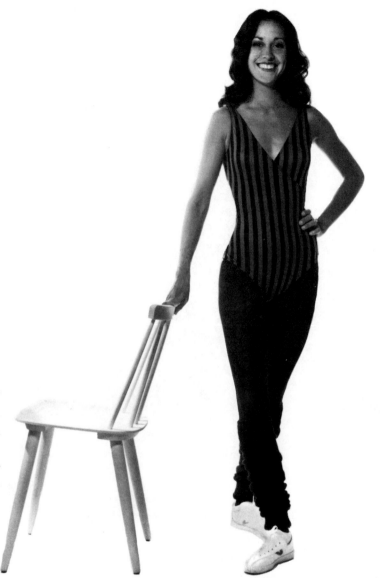

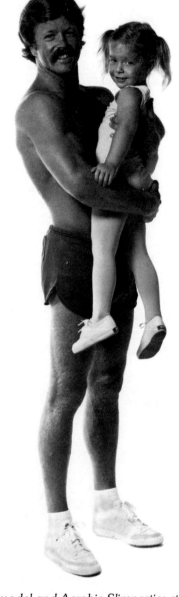

PEGGY JEMAPETE is an Aerobic Slimnastics instructor with a background in dance. Exercise has brought Peggy an inner peace and self-confidence and, as she says, "a happy, healthy heart."

BOB GILL, a professional model and Aerobic Slimnastics student, who holds a degree in physical education, has received many trophies for gymnastic competition. He says exercise helps him maintain the quality in his life. He's pictured here with little MOLLY SIMS, who, ever since she was a baby, has been watching her mother doing Aerobic Slimnastics and, as you will see, enthusiastically joins in on the exercises.

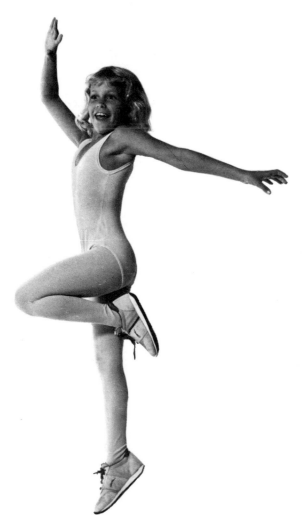

My daughter, DANA STRONG, has been energetic from the day she was born. She works out daily with the local swim team, dances, and studies gymnastics. There is such joy in her movements!

Your Basic Session

At first it will take you more than an hour to work through all five sections. That's only natural. So at the beginning—or if you ever find that you have to limit yourself to a brief workout—I suggest you follow my plan for a short, basic session. The key to making the most of your time is never to skimp on warming up and always sexercise.

WARMING UP FOR THE BIG TIME

• Do any three routines

THE BIG TIME!

• Do one routine

FANTASTIC SLIMNASTICS

• Do one standing routine

• Do one floor routine

• Do the cool-down stretch

GOOD HEALTH AND GOOD SEX

• Do every sexercise

• •

Advancing

When the exercises come easily and you feel as if you are dancing through them, when you can finish everything but the advanced routines in all five sections within an hour and feel no fatigue, only exhilaration, then you are ready to go on. If you are doing Aerobic Slimnastics three times a week for about one hour each session, you will be ready to go on in about eight weeks. But so much depends on you.

When you are ready, add the advanced exercises noted in the routines, and you may begin your second, more strenuous eight-week session. Remember to "Rest" whenever necessary and continue to note the "Carefuls."

• •

Choosing Your Music

For every Aerobic Slimnastics routine, I have suggested music that will set the tempo. Always let your music be your timer and your coach. Use these suggested selections or choose your own. Since your music will be your major motivator, allow yourself the important time to make your selections. When you are familiar with the exercises and patterns, plan several different pieces for each routine. If you are exercising three times a week, you might enjoy three different pieces for each routine for musical variety. Before you start exercising, have the records or tapes lined up, out of their cases and ready to go.

When you put your music on, really flow with the rhythm. Listen for the musical phrases, the beats and words that hang together. Your music will set the tone of your program for your body. As you exercise, let each note encourage your body to move.

I have not told you how many times to repeat

each exercise; that depends on you, your body, your fitness level today, and how frequently you do Aerobic Slimnastics. Work each exercise through a phrase of music. If the exercise calls for working both sides of your body, exercise one side through the musical phrase before you change to the other side.

While doing Aerobic Slimnastics, never stand still. If you are off the musical phrase, repeat one of the exercises. If your music ends before you finish your routine, turn your song on again. If you finish your routine before your song ends, go back to the beginning of the routine or repeat exercises within the routine.

It matters little in my fitness program if you do eight or ten leg lifts. Aerobic Slimnastics frees you forever from counting each exercise—frees you to listen to your music and your body.

Recording Your Progress

Try to schedule one hour of exercise time as often as you can. Make it your personal time, regular and undisturbed. Exercising twice a week will keep you feeling alert and energetic. Exercising three or more times a week will bring you measurable aerobic and slimnastic progress.

SLIMMING AND TRIMMING

To record your slimming and trimming, fill in the measurement chart on this page before you begin your first class. Here's how to get the most accurate measurements. Always hold the tape gently around your body at these key locations:

- Arm—around widest part of your upper arm

- Bust—across the tip

- Waist—around your waist where you wear your belt, or at the indentation that appears as you bend to the side

- Abdominals—around your hip bones and across the widest part of your tummy

- Hips—around the widest part of your buttocks and across the bottom of your leotard

- Thighs—around the widest part of your thighs about three inches down your legs

Remeasure at the end of eight weeks. The change will surprise you!

YOUR SLIMMING & TRIMMING

	WEEK 1 DATE	WEEK 8 DATE	WEEK 16 DATE
ARMS			
CHEST			
WAIST			
ABDOMEN			
HIPS			
THIGH			

TAKING YOUR PULSE

Besides a tape measure, your pulse is your most valuable fitness gauge and you carry it around with you all the time. Now's the time to learn how to take advantage of this natural gift.

Right now, while you are quietly reading this book, gently place two fingers along the side of your throat, in line with your Adam's apple, and lift your chin slightly. You will feel your pulse as your heart beats and pushes blood through the large artery in your neck. Sitting and even sleeping, your body always needs oxygen from the blood for life processes. Otherwise we could actually stop breathing in the evening—our hearts could turn in at night and start up again in the morning!

Now count your pulse for six seconds. To get your rate for a minute, add a zero to your six-second measurement. I want you to have a one-minute reading because this is how pulse measurement is discussed in popular literature. This is known as your *resting pulse*.

Now walk around the room for two minutes. Take your pulse for another six seconds. You can see how much faster your heart is beating to supply oxygen and create energy for the walking effort. Run in place until your are slightly winded. Stop and stand still while you count your pulse for six seconds. This is your *active pulse*. While standing still, you have ten seconds to count your active pulse before your heart begins to slow down and your pulse drops toward its resting state.

Wait a few seconds and count your pulse again. The second pulse will usually be lower as your heart slows to meet the reduced energy needs of your body now that you are standing still. This is your *cool-down pulse*. Again, as you become more aerobically fit, the increasing efficiency of your cardiovascular system will be reflected in a more rapid drop from the active to resting pulse rate. The pulse reading is most accurate if you time it with a watch or clock with a second hand and begin to count as soon as you stop exercising.

Now we must find a safe target for you—your *active pulse guideline*—which you can use to monitor your efforts as you work out aerobically. Begin by adjusting your goals according to your age. Subtract your age from 180. If you are 40,

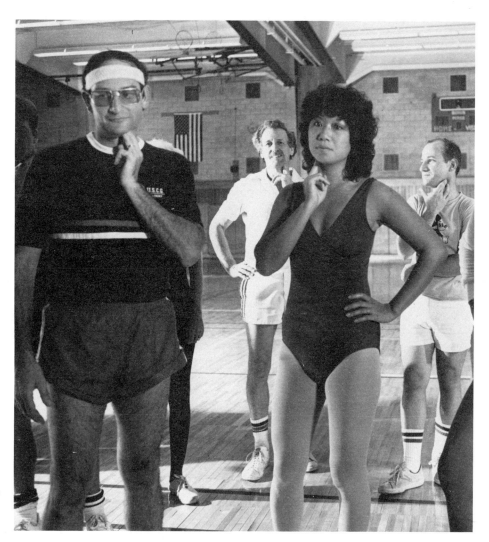

Your pulse is your most valuable fitness gauge.

your active pulse guideline would be 140 (180 − 40 = 140). The range of plus or minus ten indicated on the following Active Pulse Guideline chart will account for individual variations.

Memorize your active pulse guideline—when you are exercising aerobically, you will compare your active pulse to your active pulse guideline to monitor your progress. Your active pulse will vary depending on how much you put into the aerobic routines; your active pulse guideline will not change until your next birthday!

Take a second or two right now to record your active pulse guideline in the appropriate box in the chart entitled Your Aerobic Conditioning. You'll want to continue to use this chart when you start exercising in order to keep track of how well you're progressing. I'll be giving you directions to record your resting pulse, your active pulse, and your cool-down pulse, and showing you how to interpret that information.

Measuring the pulse is not a daily habit for most of us, and it will take some practice to get the feel of it. Practice taking your active pulse during the day after a variety of activities, and taking your resting pulse when you have been inactive for at least ten minutes. The average American resting pulse is between 70 and 80 beats per minute. Highly trained athletes Bjorn Borg and Diana Nyad have resting pulses of about 40. If your resting pulse is over 90, please see your family physician to discuss the other factors that affect pulse, such as heredity, medication, weight, blood pressure, and your life-style. As you progress with Aerobic Slimnastics, your active and resting pulse rates will drop as your heart conditions itself to deliver more oxygen with less beats per minute and your entire cardiovascular system becomes more efficient.

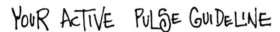

YOUR ACTIVE PULSE GUIDELINE

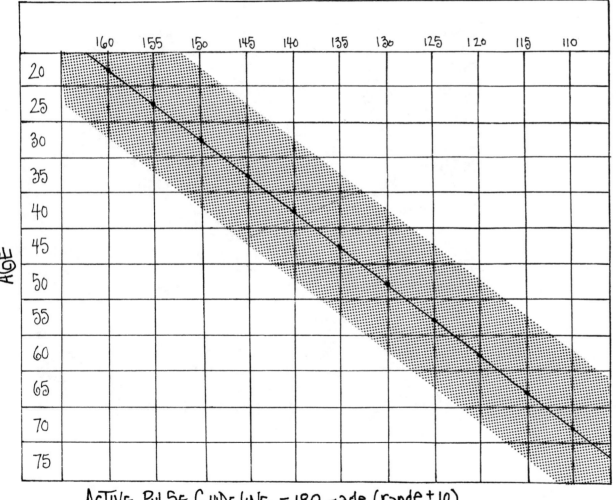

ACTIVE PULSE GUIDELINE = 180 − age (range ± 10)

YOUR AEROBIC CONDITIONING

WEEK #	YOUR RESTING PULSE (sitting & relaxing for at least 10 min.)			YOUR ACTIVE PULSE (huffing & puffing) your guideline [ ] (180 minus age)			YOUR COOL-DOWN PULSE (at end of exercise)		
	DAY 1	DAY 2	DAY 3	DAY 1	DAY 2	DAY 3	DAY 1	DAY 2	DAY 3
1									
2									
3									
4									
5									
6									
7									
8									
9									
10									
11									
12									
13									
14									
15									
16									

Dressing the Part

Comfortable exercise clothes that allow freedom of movement like shorts or warm-ups are adequate, of course. But I'd really like to see you in leotards and tights that are close fitting, warming for your muscles, and supportive of good posture. We can hide in blue jeans, dresses, or warm-ups, but a leotard keeps no secrets.

Jogging sneakers are comfortable, but if you are shopping for a sneaker specifically for Aerobic Slimnastics, look for one that gives you lateral support as well as cushioning—a sneaker designed for racquet sports or for aerobics. Leg warmers feel good and keep the leg muscles warm. Wear a warm covering like a sweat suit until you are well warmed up. An exercise mat, bath towel, rug, or blanket will keep you comfortable for floor work.

Standing Tall

Here's how you can reduce back and knee strain, relax tense shoulders, lift your bust, expand your chest, improve pelvic support for your internal organs, and tuck away five pounds without lifting a finger.

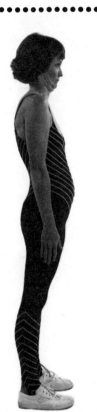 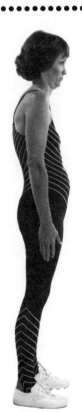 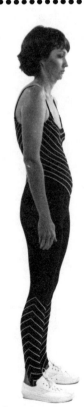 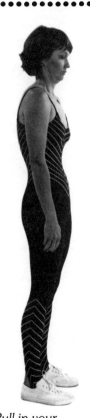 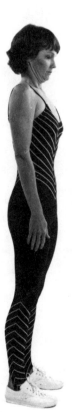 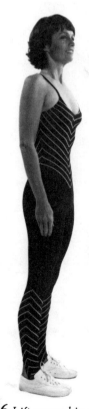

1 *Stand sideways in front of your mirror. Let everything "hang out."*

2 *Unlock your knees. Tip your pelvis back.*

3 *Tuck your buttocks under.*

4 *Pull in your abdominal muscles.*

5 *Lift your chest.*

6 *Lift your chin up and relax your shoulders.*

BEFORE　　**AFTER**

Changing your entire image may take just a few seconds and a little practice.

Extra Protection

Strong back, abdominal, and pelvic muscles—the muscles that hold you up inside and out—are extremely important to your overall health and well-being. Of these three areas, the muscles of the pelvic floor diagramed at right are often sadly ignored in exercise programs. These layered pelvic muscles are basically suspended like a hammock from the front and back of your pelvis. In our upright, human position, the downward pull of gravity, the stresses of childbirth, and the frequent increases of pressure from within our bodies make the pelvic floor prone to sagging as a hammock does. When this happens, your internal organs slip down, giving you considerable discomfort when you are active. It may be difficult for you to prevent urine leakage. You may be uncomfortable making love. Strong abdominal muscles working together with the pelvic muscles keep your internal organs supported, protect your lower back, and contribute significantly to good feelings of being physically able.

Happily for us, abdominal, pelvic, and lower back muscles respond well and quickly to a brief but regular routine of concentrated exercise. The "Extra Protection" exercises on the following pages provide just such a routine. The muscles in the middle are so crucial to your overall fitness that I want you to sexercise ten minutes *every day* no matter what, just before you go to bed and as soon as you get up in the morning, until these exercises are as routine as combing your hair.

To use the Sexercises as part of your complete Aerobic Slimnastics program, see pages 182–186.

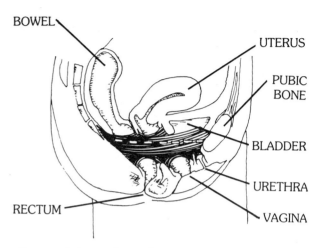

Strong abdominal muscles support internal organs.

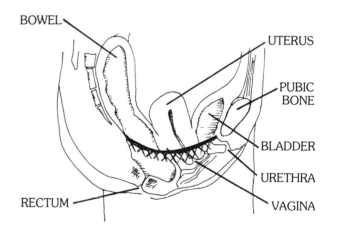

Weak abdominal muscles let organs sag.

Sexercises

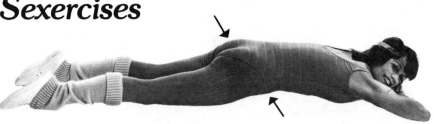
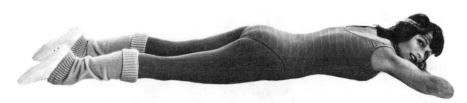

1 Pelvic Push Lie prone on the floor with your head resting on your arms. Tighten your seat. Pull your buttocks together and pull in your abdominal muscles. Your pelvis will tip under and there will be a little space under your abdomen. Hold everything in a "Kegel" as Lamaze prenatal classes recommend—that is, as if you were looking for the restroom in a crowded theater.

2 Relax all your muscles. When the Pelvic Push becomes second nature, you can practice it anywhere standing up by tightening when a meeting is boring, when waiting for stop lights to change, or when doing dishes. Never a wasted moment!

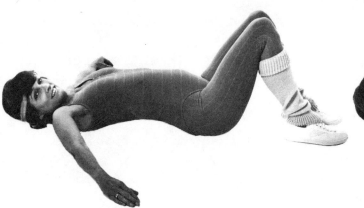
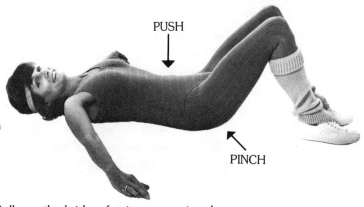

PUSH

PINCH

1 Bridge Lie on your back with knees bent and feet flat on the floor about 18 inches apart. Keeping your shoulders and buttocks tight to the floor, arch the small of your back slightly to make a little bridge.

2 Collapse the bridge, forcing your spine down. Tilt your pelvis under and tighten your buttocks. Tighten everything. Then relax. Repeat the entire sequence several times.

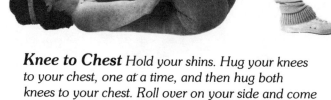

Knee to Chest Hold your shins. Hug your knees to your chest, one at a time, and then hug both knees to your chest. Roll over on your side and come up on your hands and knees.

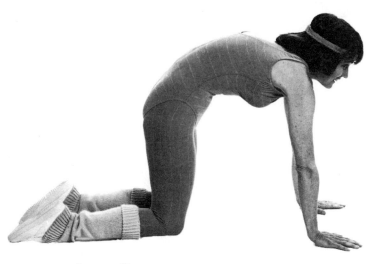

Angry Cat *On your hands and knees, keeping your arms straight, arch your back like an angry Halloween cat. Pull everything in and tighten your abdominal muscles. Hold for three counts while your neck is relaxed and you're looking down.*

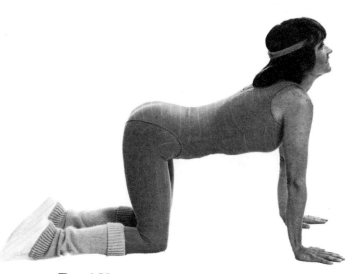

Tired Horse *Sag like a tired horse, keeping your elbows straight. Relax your abdominal muscles, lift your head, and smile. Repeat several times.*

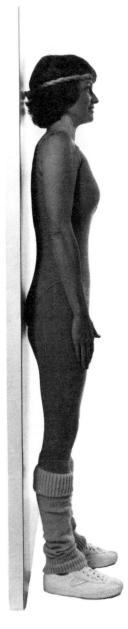

1 Standing Pelvic Tilt *To relieve tension or lower back pain, stand with your back against a wall. Place your feet several inches from the wall, with your head, shoulders, and buttocks touching the wall and your knees relaxed.*

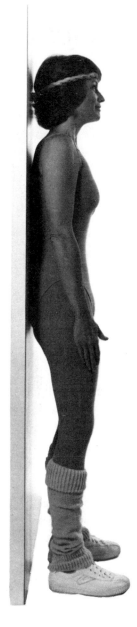

2 *Pull your abdominal muscles in and pinch your buttocks together strongly. The small of your back will flatten to the wall. Hold for ten counts. Relax and repeat several times. Your body will feel refreshed.*

Using Weights

Wrist weights can complement each exercise in your Aerobic Slimnastics program, further developing your strength and increasing your aerobic conditioning. The best weights are designed with removable cylindrical weights, which can be inserted in pockets in a lightweight material that you wrap around your wrist and secure firmly with a velcro fastener or a clasp.

Ankle weights may increase your risk of back strain, so for Aerobic Slimnastics, leave your weights on your wrist. Begin with minimum weights, increasing gradually as your strength increases. Keep the weight challenging but manageable so you can maintain full aerobic movement.

Arranging Your Space

Your exercise space should be as large as possible. Adjust the furniture so you have room to kick your legs to the front, side, and back, swing your arms, move to the right and left and clap your hands over your head. The room should be a comfortable temperature and free from drafts. When setting the temperature, it is far better to be on the warm side than to have the room too cold. The warm air will help warm your muscles and keep you perspiring freely.

Put a "Do Not Disturb" sign on the door, turn off the phone, put the baby to bed, send the children outside (or put them in leotards, too!), put your work away, and begin. You have a date with yourself.

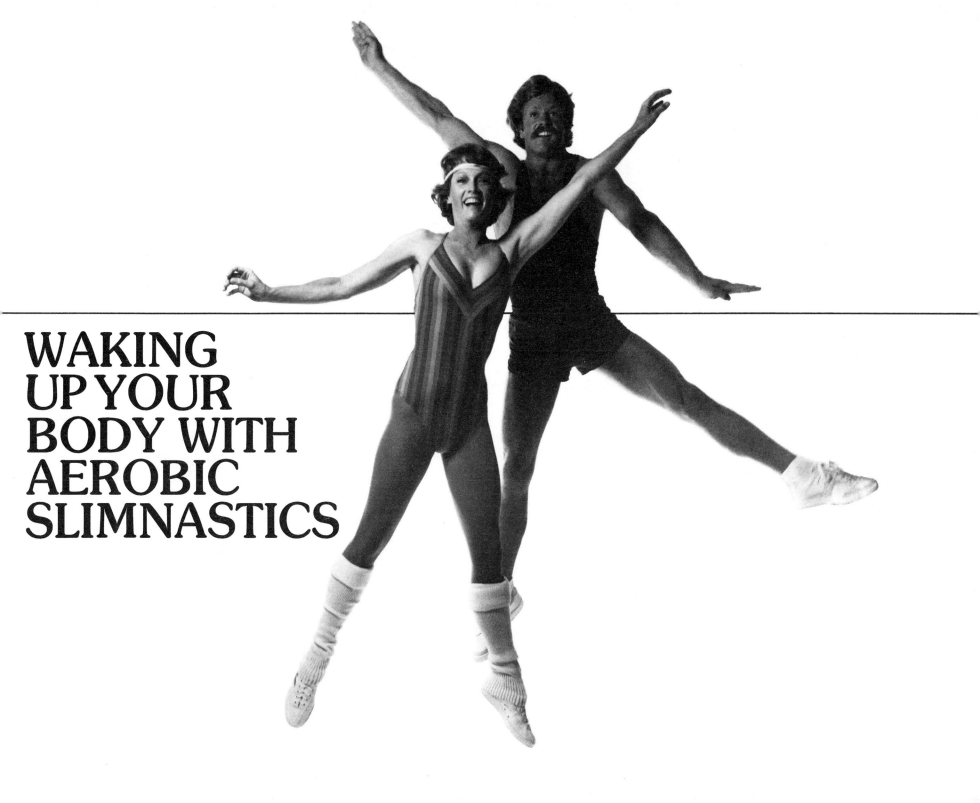

WAKING UP YOUR BODY WITH AEROBIC SLIMNASTICS

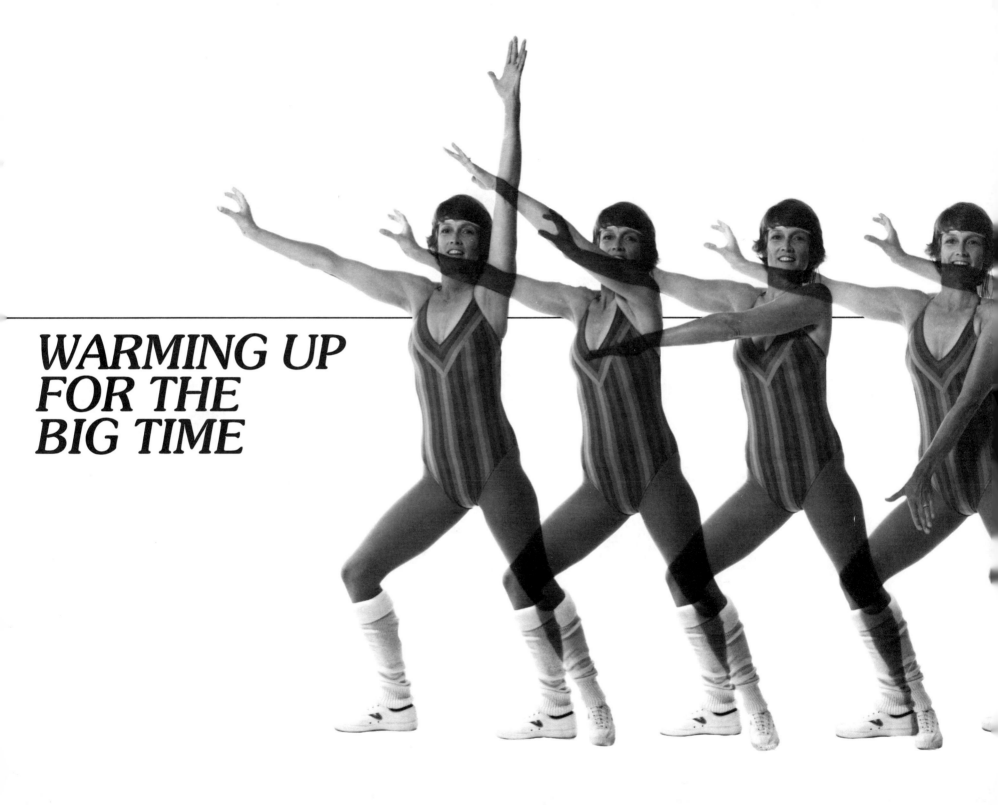

WARMING UP
FOR THE
BIG TIME

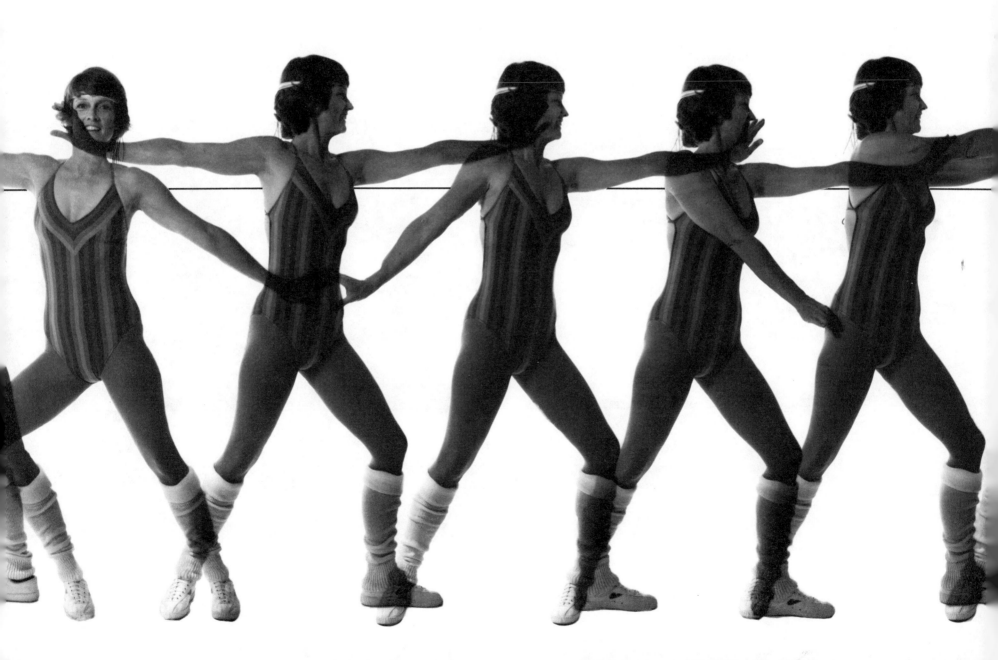

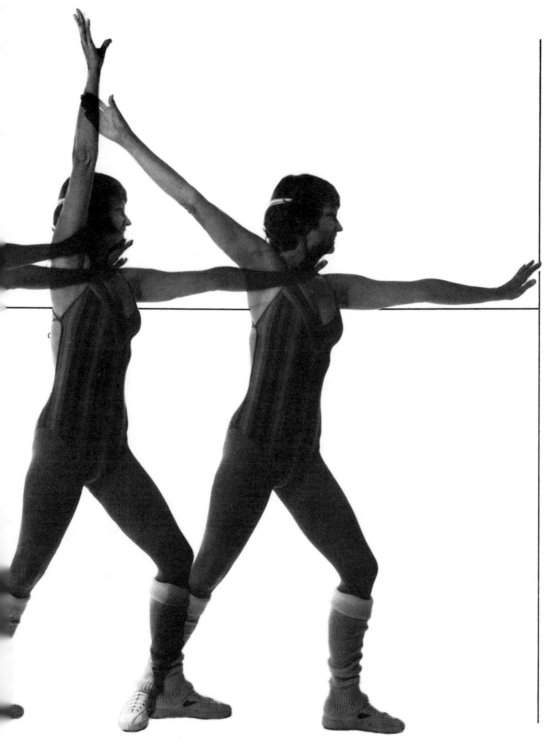

CONTENTS

*First and most important is the warm-up routine. The exercises
in this section will warm up your muscles by increasing the blood
and oxygen supply to them. Your muscle fibers will become
more flexible and more resistant to injury. You will stretch all the
muscle groups as you practice slowly many of the exercises
that are repeated later in the program at a different tempo.
The warm-up is your body's opportunity to get ready for the fun.*

Getting Started

Feel your music call to your muscles to stretch and warm them. Set your warm-up patterns to the musical phrases. Repeat each pattern until you are comfortable with it. If you are off the musical phrase a little, repeat part of the pattern.

The music should remind you of a colorful sunrise or a sleek cat waking up and stretching.

Suggestions:
1. "Weekend," Barry Manilow, *Greatest Hits,* Arista Records
2. "Always on My Mind," Willie Nelson, *Always on My Mind,* Columbia Records
3. Titles from the original soundtrack of *Chariots of Fire,* Polydor Records

CAREFUL
Do not bounce through the warm-up exercises. Enjoy a long, slow stretch in each routine.

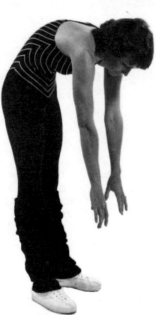
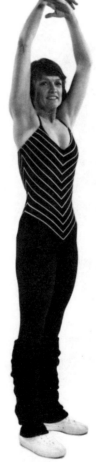
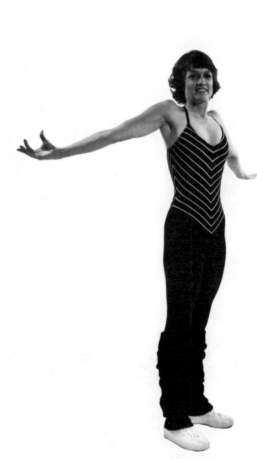

1 ***Pull up*** As the music begins, stand with your feet pointing forward and placed comfortably at about shoulder-width apart. Bend over at the waist. Do not bounce or push—let gravity do the work. Keep your knees straight—not locked, but straight.

2 Pull up slowly from the waist with rounded back, tuck your buttocks under, and tilt your pelvis back.

3 Continue to pull up until you're standing tall, arms overhead.

4 Finish by making a big circle, dropping and crossing your arms in front of your body. As you bring your arms back up, lift your rib cage off your waist, stretching back. Open your arms wide apart and *enjoy this luxurious stretch.*

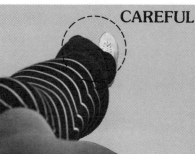

CAREFUL   **Never**
As you lunge look down your thigh and off your knee, you should not be able to see your leading foot. If you can, your foot is awkwardly twisted and you are resting precariously off balance and possibly endangering your ankle and knee.

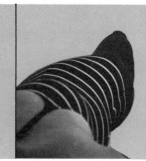

Always
If your feet are perpendicular to each other as you are lunging, you will not be able to see the toes of your lunging foot as you look down your thigh, and you will be safely positioned.

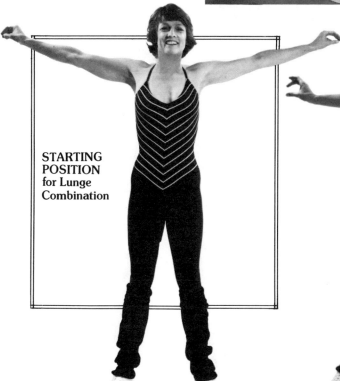

STARTING POSITION for Lunge Combination

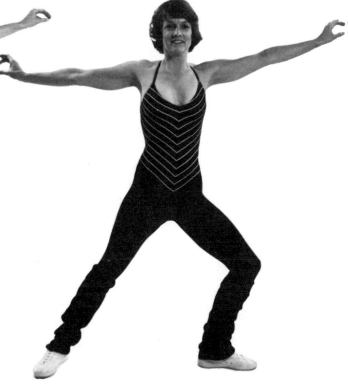

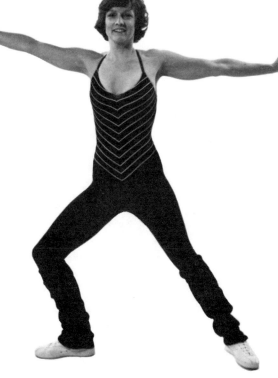

LUNGE COMBINATION

Stand with your feet slightly apart and arms out at shoulder level. When the directions say "Step out to the right," I'm pictured stepping to the left, but remember the photographs are intended to be your mirror image.

1 *Lunge* Step out to the right. Be sure your feet are perpendicular to each other. Tuck your abdominal muscles in and your buttocks under. Center your shoulders over your hips. Bend your right knee. When you look down your thigh, you should not see your toes. Feel your right thigh muscle warming. Gently straighten your right knee and return to starting position.

2 Lunge to the left. Be sure your feet are perpendicular to each other by looking down your thigh. Bend your left knee as you lunge and then gently straighten. Return to starting position.

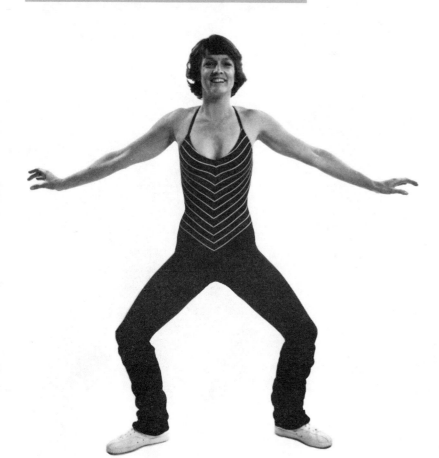

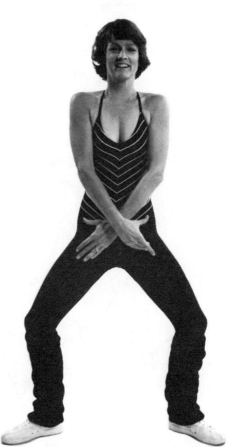

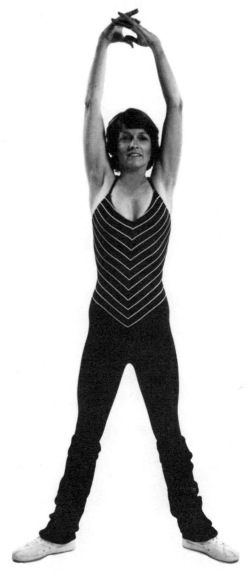

1 *Deep Knee Bend* Turn your feet so that your toes are pointing out. Keeping your feet flat, imagine that some of your weight is on the little toes. Bend your knees over your toes, keeping your back straight, abdominal muscles tight, and buttocks tucked under.

2 As you bend your knees, let your thighs do the work.

3 As you come up, straighten but do not lock your knees, and add a Big Arm Circle.

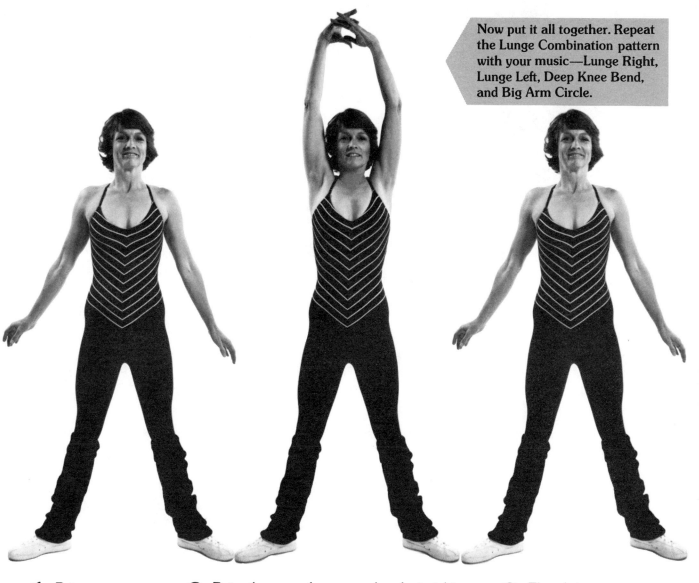

Now put it all together. Repeat the Lunge Combination pattern with your music—Lunge Right, Lunge Left, Deep Knee Bend, and Big Arm Circle.

Big Arm Circle This basic exercise is essential to your warm-up: It stretches your arm, shoulder, upper back, and chest muscles. Use Big Arm Circles whenever you like throughout your warm-up. If you finish your warm-ups before your music ends, continue to do Big Arm Circles. Remember, whenever the music is playing it's your cue to exercise.

1 Bring your arms down and cross to circle in front of your body.

2 Raise them up above your head, stretching your arms behind your ears as you continue reaching behind you. As you stretch up, really lift your rib cage, pull in your abdominal muscles, and tighten your buttocks. *Think very tall and breathe.*

3 Then bring your arms down again.

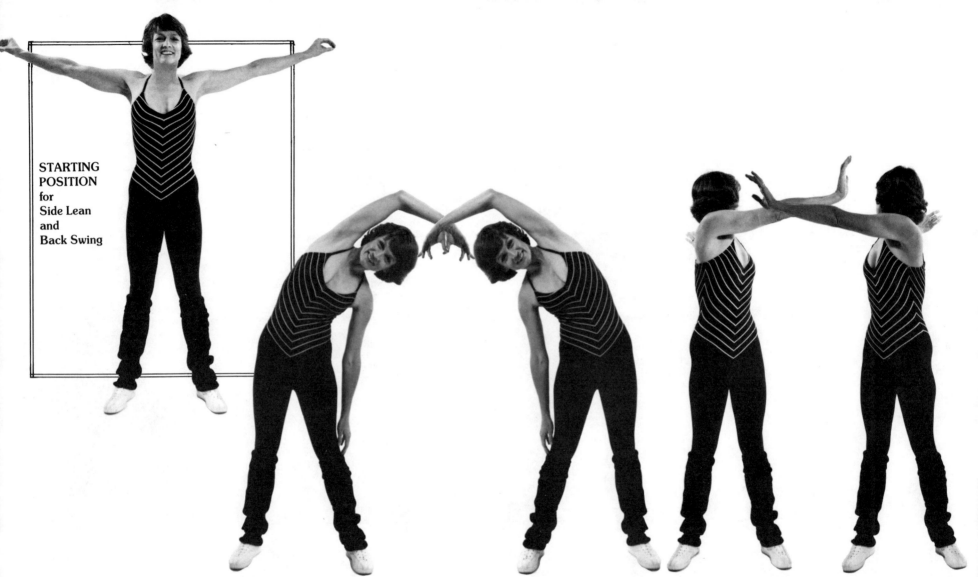

WAIST WARMER
Stand tall, holding your arms out at shoulder level, feet facing forward and comfortably apart. Pull your abdominal muscles in and tuck your buttocks under.

1 *Side Lean* Slide your hand down the side of your leg as you lift your opposite shoulder and stretch your opposite arm over your head. Feel the wonderful long stretch along your rib cage and waist.

2 Alternate sides and remember to *stretch slowly*—do not bounce.

1 *Back Swing* Keep your arms at shoulder level. Swing your upper body gently toward the back, watching your back hand as you swing.

2 Set up an easy Back Swing to alternate sides with no bouncing.

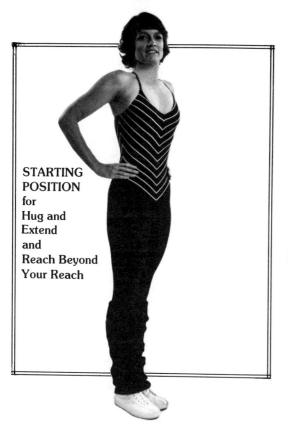

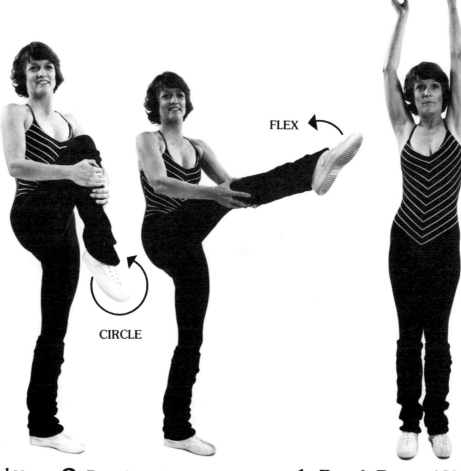

CIRCLE

FLEX

EXTENSION STRETCH

Pull your abdominal muscles in and tighten your buttocks. Stand tall.

1 ***Hug and Extend*** Hug your shin as you bring your right knee in above your waist. Circle your foot. Feel the muscles along your shin working.

2 Extend your leg, pointing your toes. Flex your foot, and slowly lower it. Shaky balance? Tighten your buttocks and watch a fixed spot on the wall. Repeat with the left leg.

1 ***Reach Beyond Your Reach*** Stand, feet comfortably apart, with both arms over your head. Reach Beyond Your Reach with one arm at a time.

2 Alternate one arm higher than the other to the beat of the music. End with a Big Arm Circle.

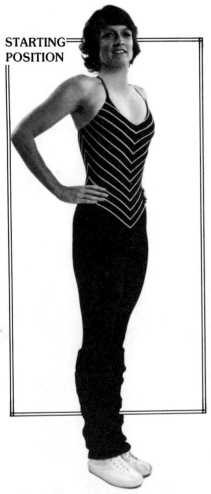

STARTING POSITION

STRIDING SALUTE
Stand with your feet together and your hands on your hips.

Stride Forward
On a lunge your feet are perpendicular with the lunging knee bent. On a stride your feet are parallel with the striding knee bent. *Stride* forward on your right leg, keeping your feet parallel. Bend your forward knee. Feel the stretch in the muscles along the back of your leg.

Hand to Cheek
Bring the back of your right hand to your cheek, keeping your elbow high, and . . .

1 Circle Way Back
. . . circle your right arm up and behind you.

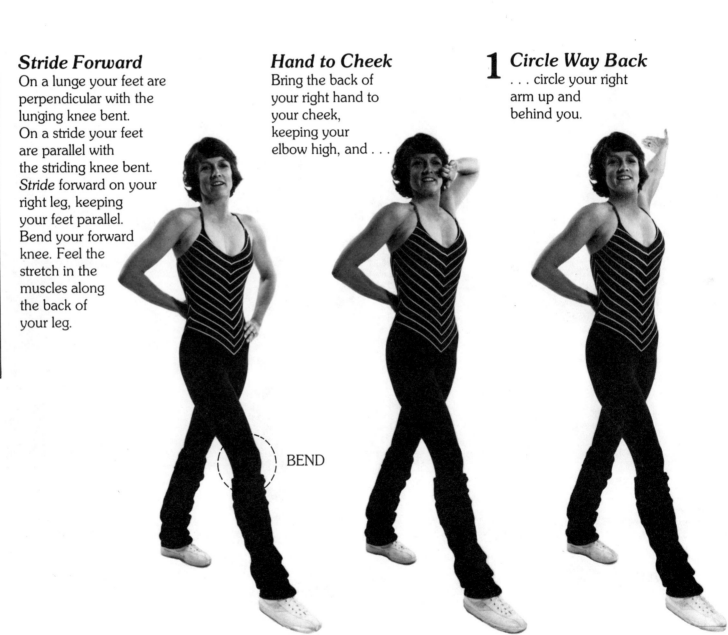

BEND

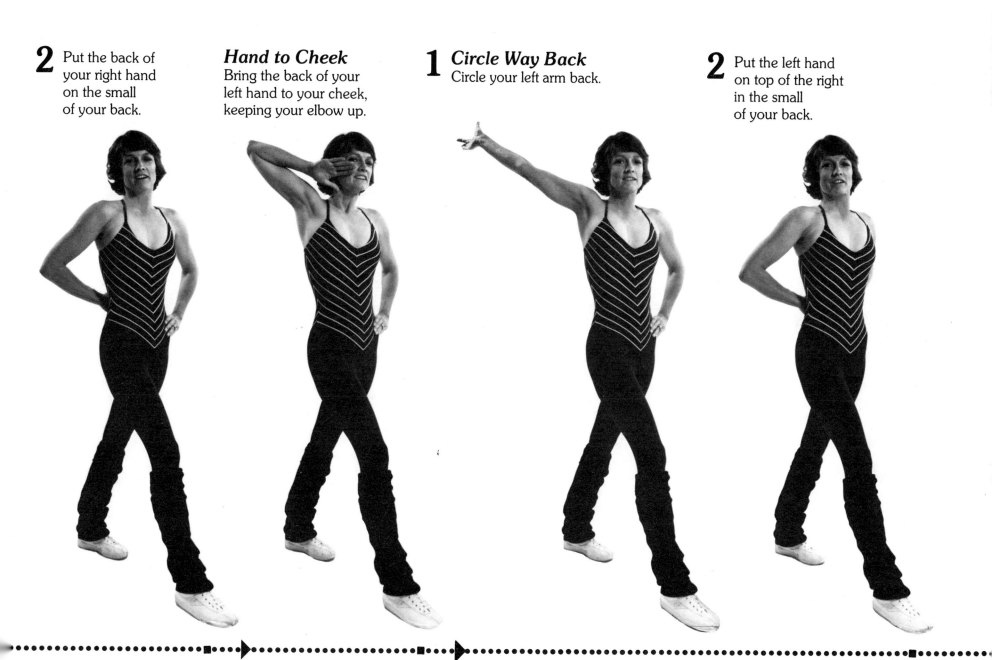

2 Put the back of your right hand on the small of your back.

Hand to Cheek
Bring the back of your left hand to your cheek, keeping your elbow up.

1 ***Circle Way Back***
Circle your left arm back.

2 Put the left hand on top of the right in the small of your back.

Flat Back Stretch

Bend over your striding leg from your waist, keeping your back flat and the striding knee bent. Keep your chin and shoulders up as you stretch the muscles of your lower back.

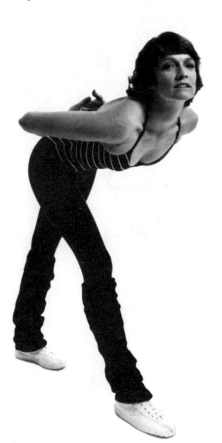

Heel Stretch

Stand up and gently bounce the heel of your back foot twice, stretching out the back of your leg.

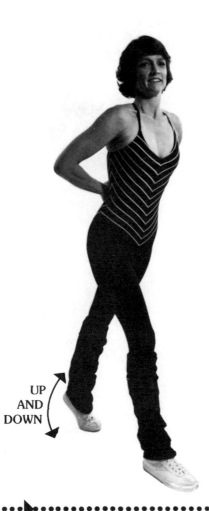

UP
AND
DOWN

1 ### Knee Stretch

Shift your weight to your right leg. Bring your back knee up in front of you. Flex your foot. Again feel the stretch.

FLEX

2 Put your foot down next to your standing foot.

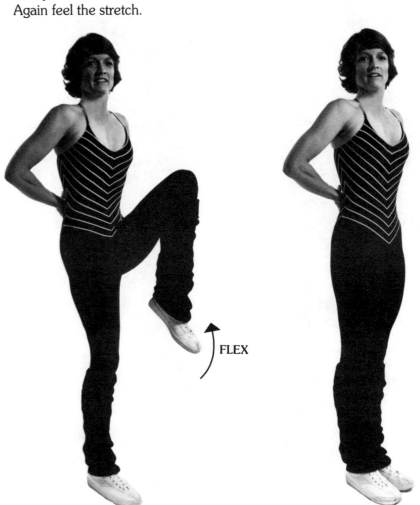

Hands to Cheeks

Bring the backs of both
hands to your cheeks
and circle your
arms back.

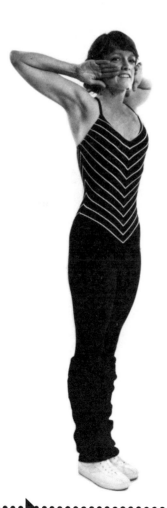

Circle Way Back

Feel the pull in your
shoulders and upper arms.

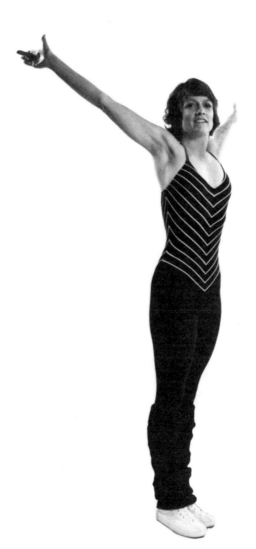

*Really stretch!
You look wonderful!*

NOW...
Repeat the entire
Striding Salute on
the left side,
striding forward on
your left leg.

1 *Prayer Stretch*
Stand tall with your hands clasped in front of you.

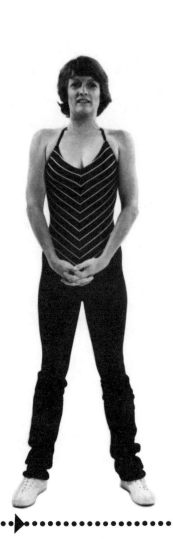

2 Raise your clasped hands to the right. Turn your "prayer" hands inside out and stretch. Return to position 1.

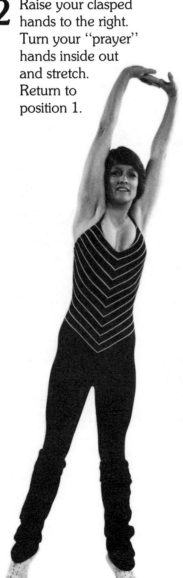

3 Center your arms over your head. Turn your "prayer" inside out and stretch. Return to position 1.

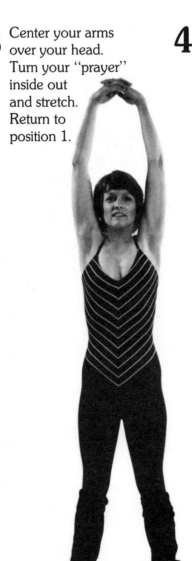

4 Raise your "prayer" arms to the left. Turn your hands inside out and stretch. *Your arms, hands, and even your fingers will feel so good.*

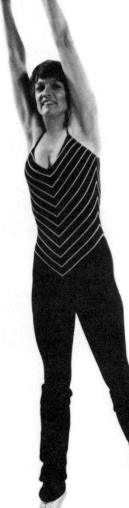

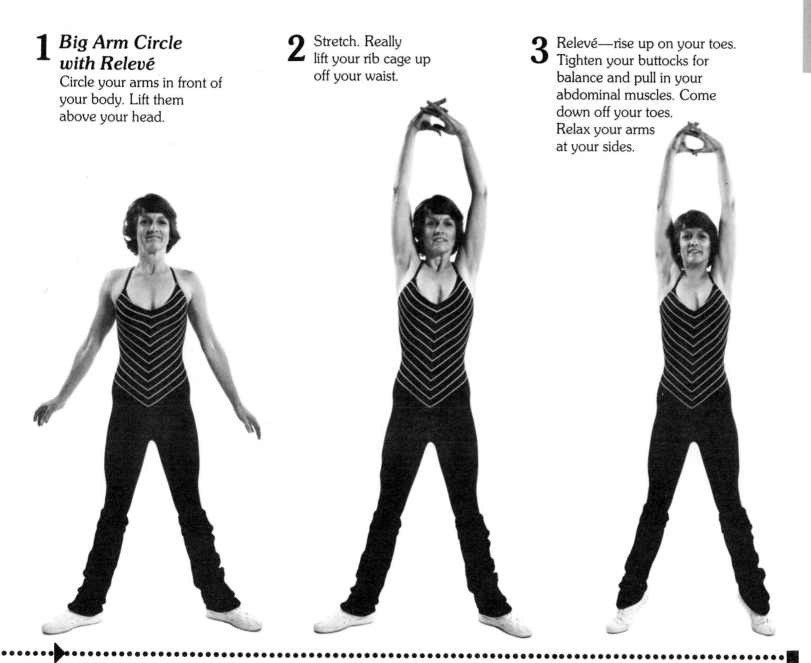

1 ***Big Arm Circle
with Relevé***
Circle your arms in front of
your body. Lift them
above your head.

2 Stretch. Really
lift your rib cage up
off your waist.

3 Relevé—rise up on your toes.
Tighten your buttocks for
balance and pull in your
abdominal muscles. Come
down off your toes.
Relax your arms
at your sides.

*You are
ready now
to pick up
your pace
aerobically.*

Walking Warm-up

Walking is your body's best friend. It is a total warm-up from head to toe. By gradually increasing your pace you can warm up your large-muscle groups and your cardiovascular system, too.
You will be walking through many of the exercises that you will use in the more aerobic routines later on in the book. Walk in a circle, changing from one pattern to the next as your musical phrases change.
Let this lighthearted routine flow with your music.
If you do not have room for a circle, do the patterns walking in place.

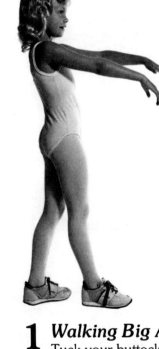
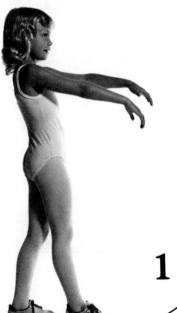
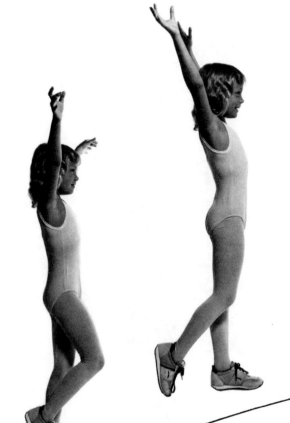
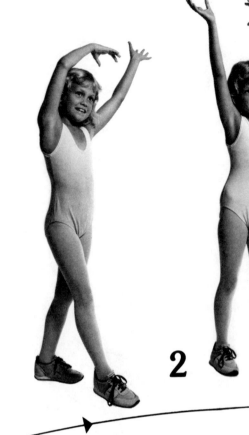

1

2

Keep moving

1 ***Walking Big Arm Circles***
Tuck your buttocks under, pull your abdominals in, lift your rib cage off your waist, hold your shoulders back, and lift chest and chin up. *You look terrific.*

Start walking. Put your heel down gently and roll off the ball of your foot. Bring your arms up and around and back by your ears, lifting your rib cage in a Big Arm Circle.

2 ***Willows*** Keep walking. Lift your rib cage off your waist, and reach and sway from side to side like a willow tree in the wind.

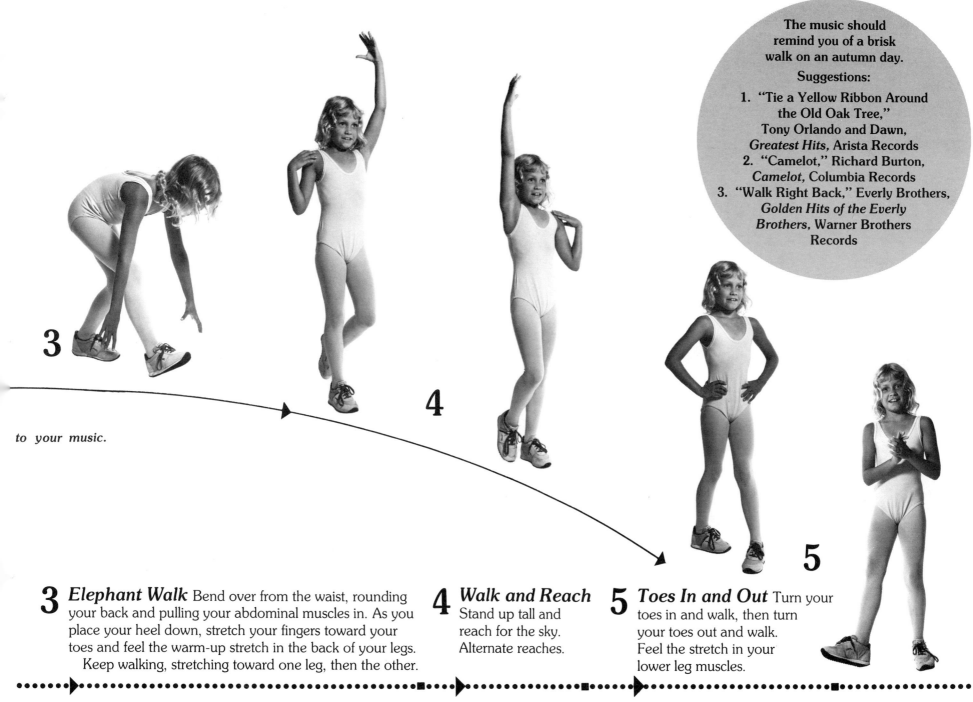

3

to your music.

4

5

3 *Elephant Walk* Bend over from the waist, rounding your back and pulling your abdominal muscles in. As you place your heel down, stretch your fingers toward your toes and feel the warm-up stretch in the back of your legs. Keep walking, stretching toward one leg, then the other.

4 *Walk and Reach* Stand up tall and reach for the sky. Alternate reaches.

5 *Toes In and Out* Turn your toes in and walk, then turn your toes out and walk. Feel the stretch in your lower leg muscles.

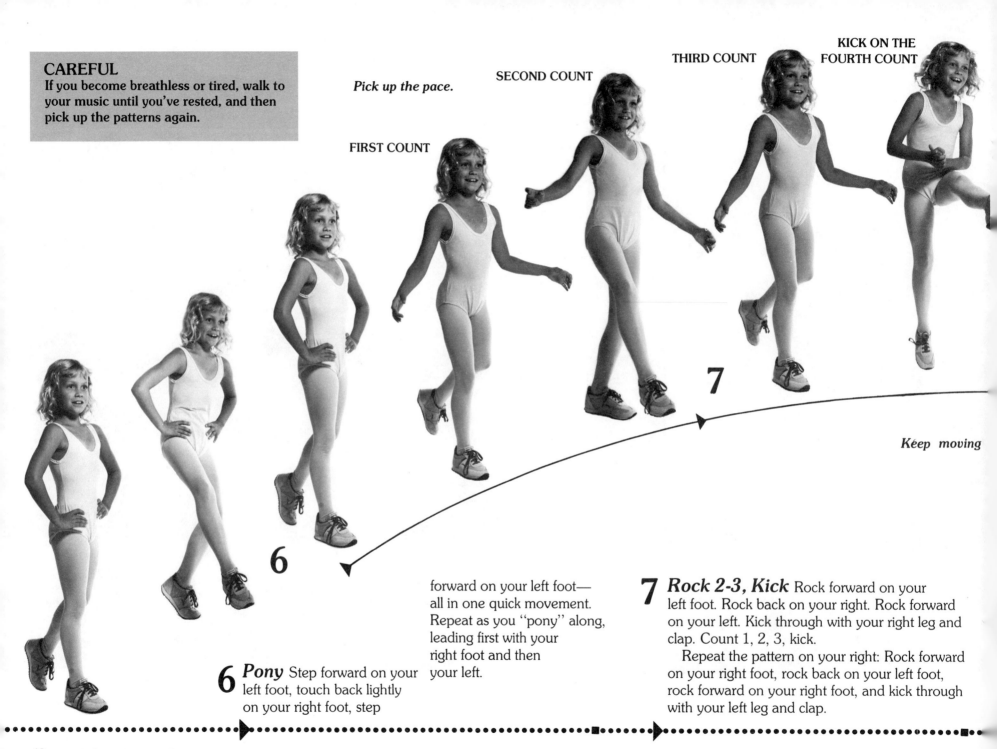

THIRD COUNT

SECOND COUNT

Pick up the pace.

FIRST COUNT

CAREFUL
If you become breathless or tired, walk to your music until you've rested, and then pick up the patterns again.

7

Keep moving

6

forward on your left foot—all in one quick movement. Repeat as you "pony" along, leading first with your right foot and then your left.

6 *Pony* Step forward on your left foot, touch back lightly on your right foot, step

7 *Rock 2-3, Kick* Rock forward on your left foot. Rock back on your right. Rock forward on your left. Kick through with your right leg and clap. Count 1, 2, 3, kick.

Repeat the pattern on your right: Rock forward on your right foot, rock back on your left foot, rock forward on your right foot, and kick through with your left leg and clap.

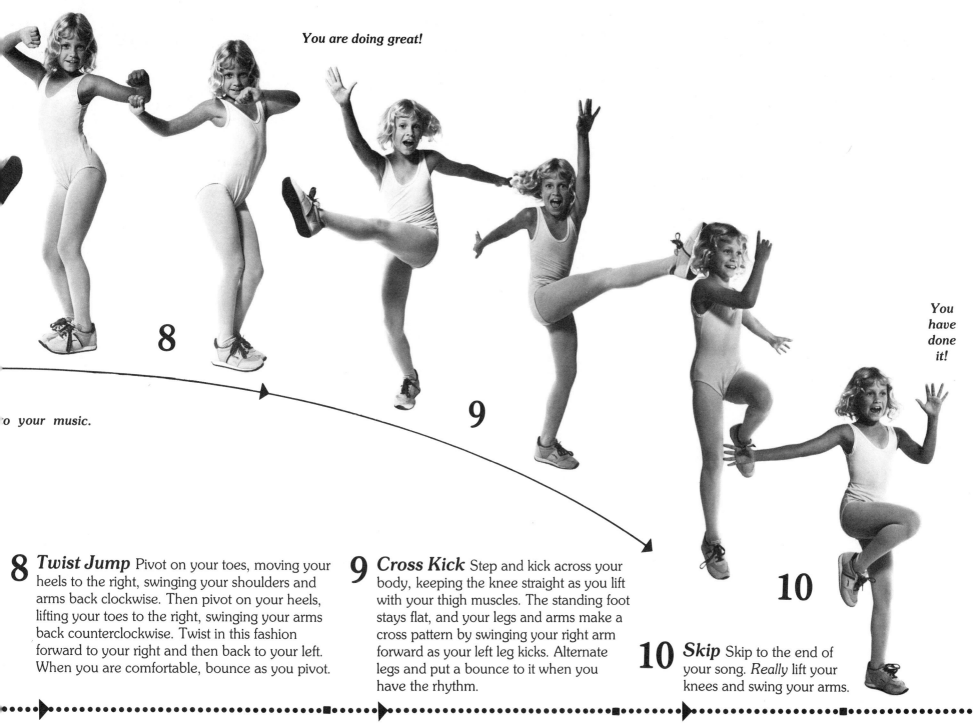

You are doing great!

o your music.

8

9

You have done it!

10

8 *Twist Jump* Pivot on your toes, moving your heels to the right, swinging your shoulders and arms back clockwise. Then pivot on your heels, lifting your toes to the right, swinging your arms back counterclockwise. Twist in this fashion forward to your right and then back to your left. When you are comfortable, bounce as you pivot.

9 *Cross Kick* Step and kick across your body, keeping the knee straight as you lift with your thigh muscles. The standing foot stays flat, and your legs and arms make a cross pattern by swinging your right arm forward as your left leg kicks. Alternate legs and put a bounce to it when you have the rhythm.

10 *Skip* Skip to the end of your song. *Really* lift your knees and swing your arms.

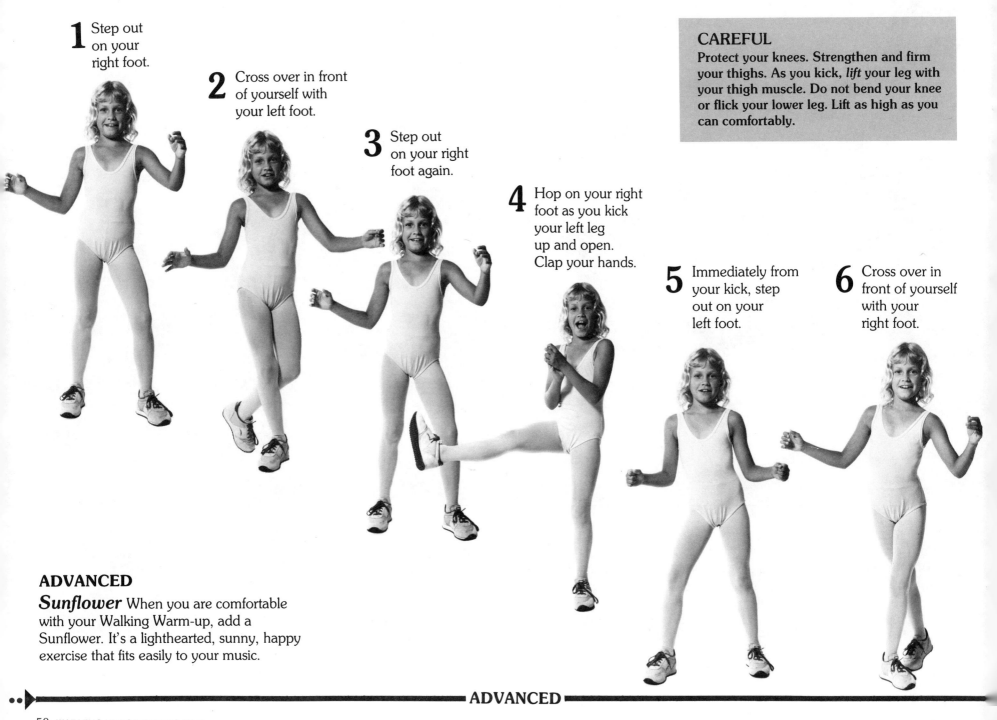

1 Step out on your right foot.

2 Cross over in front of yourself with your left foot.

3 Step out on your right foot again.

4 Hop on your right foot as you kick your left leg up and open. Clap your hands.

5 Immediately from your kick, step out on your left foot.

6 Cross over in front of yourself with your right foot.

ADVANCED

Sunflower When you are comfortable with your Walking Warm-up, add a Sunflower. It's a lighthearted, sunny, happy exercise that fits easily to your music.

◆◆▶ ━━━━━━━━━━━ **ADVANCED** ━━━━━━━━━━━

You are doing the Sunflower.
Feel the movement and the rhythm
of the exercise within yourself.
You are "dancing," and you may
even feel like singing.

7 Step out on your left foot again.

8 Hop on your left foot as you kick up and open.

9 Immediately set your kicking leg down to the right.

10 Cross over with your left.

11 Step on your right foot again.

12 Hop, kick, and clap.

Repeat the Sunflower until you feel comfortable with the steps. Either walk this exercise out slowly and gently kick, or jog through the steps and really lift your leg. Adjust the exercise to the beat of your music.

ADVANCED

Stretching Out

With this routine you will thoroughly warm up your
leg muscles so that you will be ready to dance.
You will need something to hold on to
for balance—not for support.
Use a ballet bar, a sturdy
chair, or a wall.

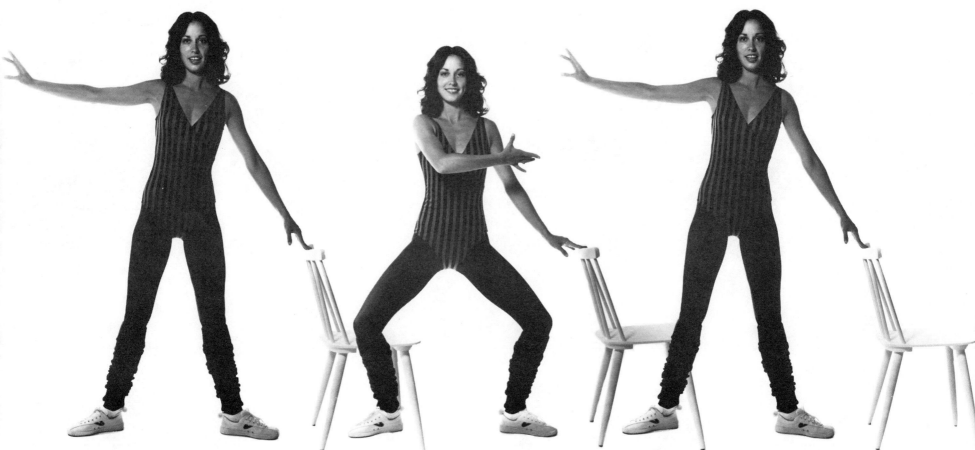

1 *Deep Knee Bend* Keep your back
straight, buttocks tucked under, your
abdominal muscles in. Keep your feet flat,
shoulder-width apart, and pointing out.

2 Bend your knees out over
your toes. *Think thighs.*

3 Repeat several knee bends through
the introduction of your music.

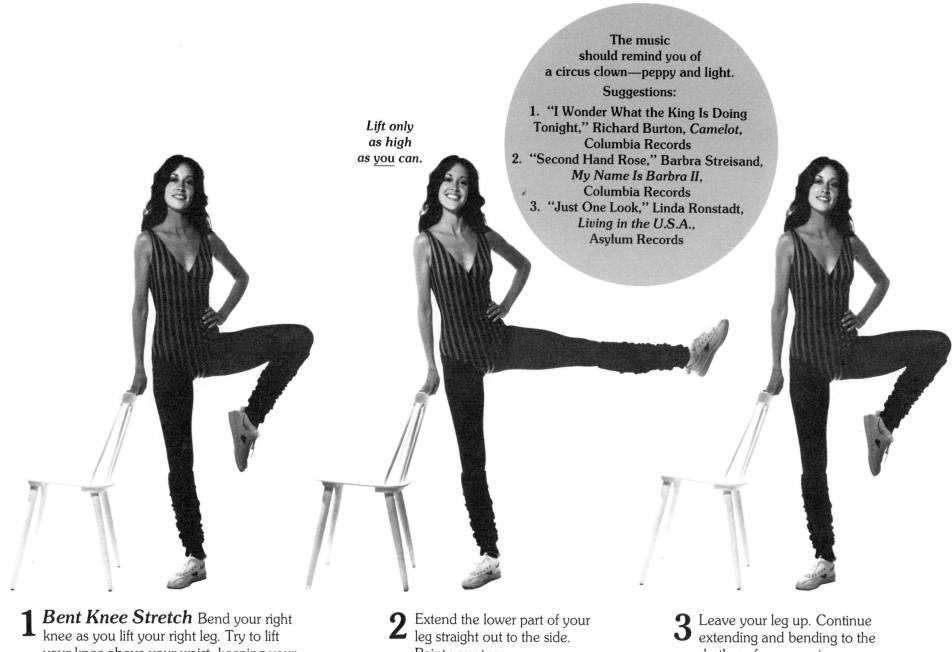

*Lift only
as high
as <u>you</u> can.*

The music
should remind you of
a circus clown—peppy and light.

Suggestions:

1. "I Wonder What the King Is Doing Tonight," Richard Burton, *Camelot,* Columbia Records
2. "Second Hand Rose," Barbra Streisand, *My Name Is Barbra II,* Columbia Records
3. "Just One Look," Linda Ronstadt, *Living in the U.S.A.,* Asylum Records

1 ***Bent Knee Stretch*** Bend your right knee as you lift your right leg. Try to lift your knee above your waist, keeping your lifted leg perpendicular to your body.

2 Extend the lower part of your leg straight out to the side. Point your toes.

3 Leave your leg up. Continue extending and bending to the rhythm of your music.

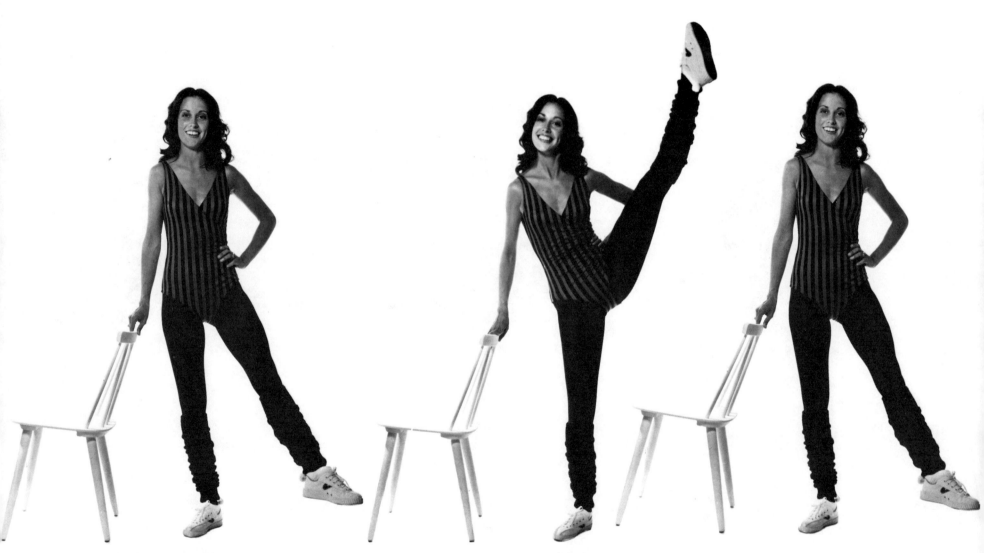

1 ***Diagonal Lift*** Point your toe and lift your leg diagonally in line with your shoulder.

2 Do not fling from the knee. *Lift,* using your thigh muscle, and only go up as high as is comfortable for you.

1 ***Side Leg Lift*** Flex your foot. Turn it perpendicular to your body and lift.

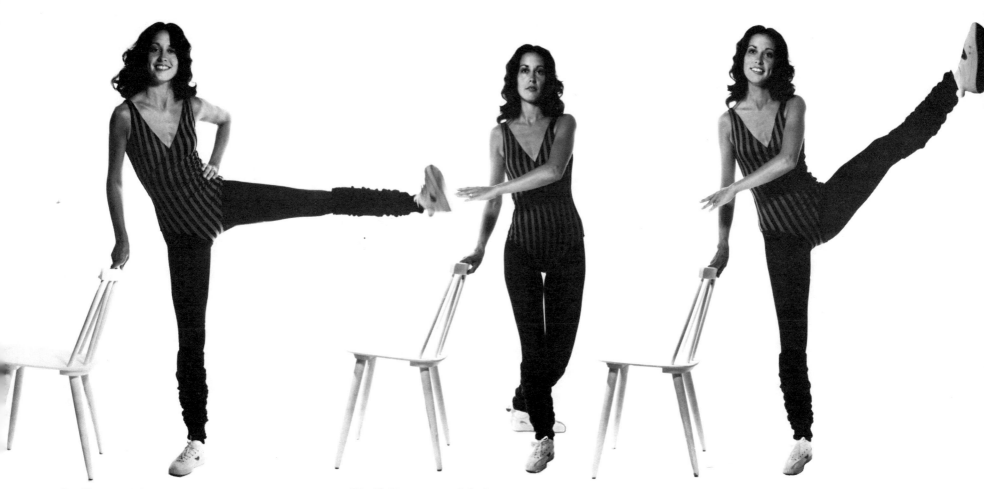

2 Be careful not to throw your leg. *Lift* with your thigh and buttocks muscles. Work with your music.

1 *Full Diagonal Lift* Bend your knees slightly, placing your right (outside) foot back. Notice the placement of the arm.

2 Lift your back leg to the front in a diagonally open kick. Keep your arm position. Lower your leg, and continue to bend and lift with your music.

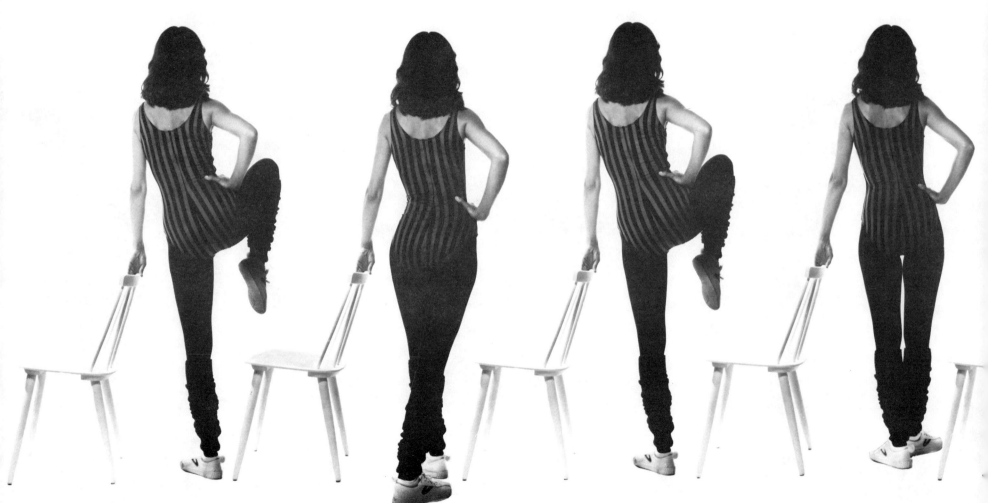

You can see the foot placement that is important in this pattern.

1 ***Strut*** Bend your knee as you lift it up above your waist, keeping your knee pointed out from your body on a diagonal.

2 Place your foot down behind your standing leg. Be sure your heels are down.

3 Lift your knee up again.

4 Lower your foot and place it in front of your standing leg. Repeat the strut to your music.

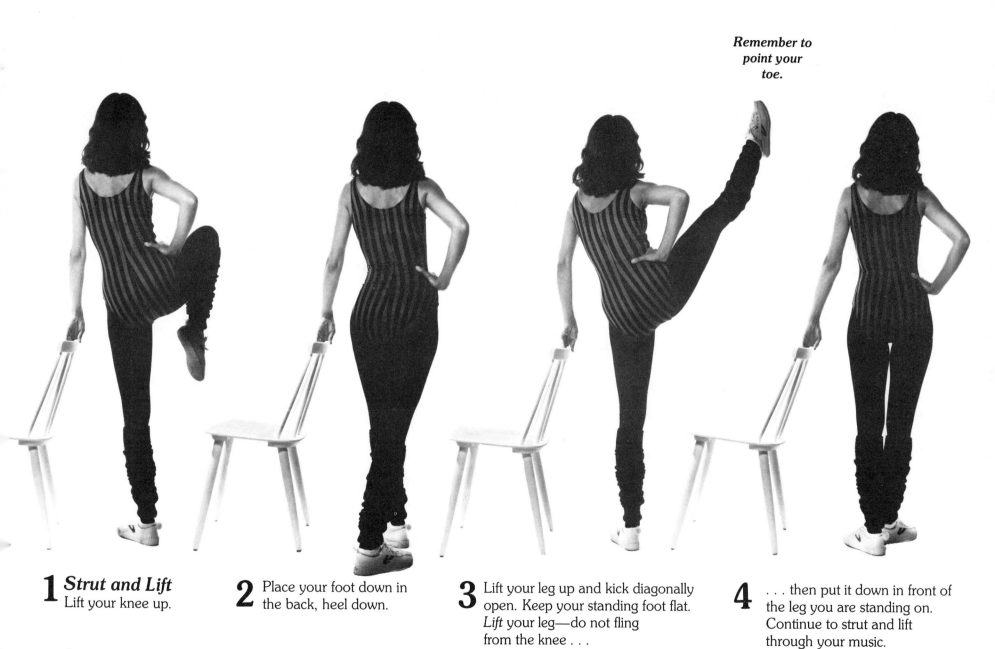

Remember to point your toe.

1 ***Strut and Lift*** Lift your knee up.

2 Place your foot down in the back, heel down.

3 Lift your leg up and kick diagonally open. Keep your standing foot flat. *Lift* your leg—do not fling from the knee . . .

4 . . . then put it down in front of the leg you are standing on. Continue to strut and lift through your music.

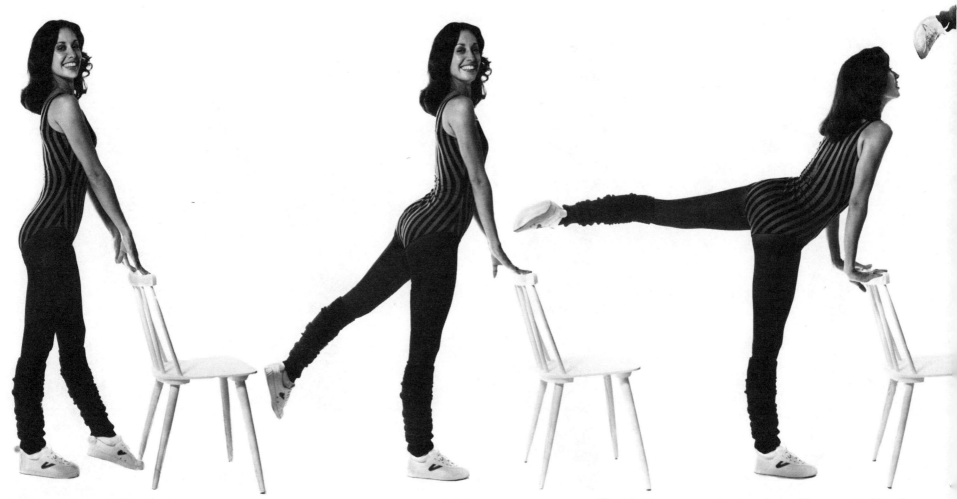

1 *Back Leg Lift* Turn and face into your support, holding it with both hands. Chin up and elbows straight.

2 Stretch your left leg out in back, pointing your toes.

3 Height is not important here. You are looking for the stretch in the legs, abdominal muscles, buttocks, and lower back. Lift and lower your leg through a phrase of music. Then repeat Back Leg Lift using your right leg.

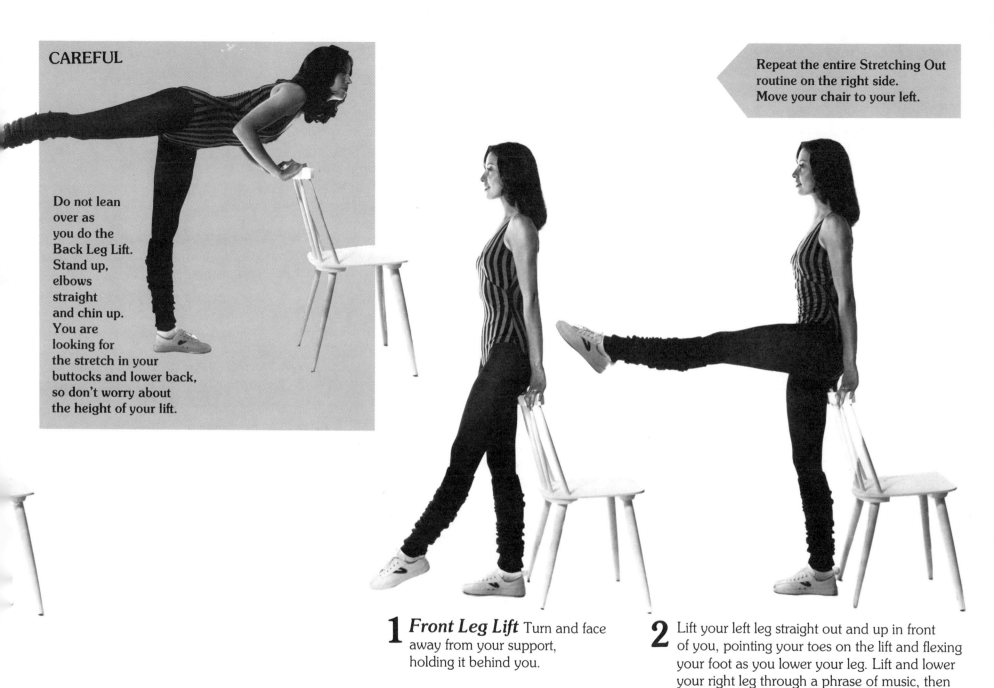

CAREFUL

Do not lean over as you do the Back Leg Lift. Stand up, elbows straight and chin up. You are looking for the stretch in your buttocks and lower back, so don't worry about the height of your lift.

Repeat the entire Stretching Out routine on the right side. Move your chair to your left.

1 *Front Leg Lift* Turn and face away from your support, holding it behind you.

2 Lift your left leg straight out and up in front of you, pointing your toes on the lift and flexing your foot as you lower your leg. Lift and lower your right leg through a phrase of music, then change and lift your other leg.

Loving Yourself

Be good to yourself! With this warm-up routine, tighten and tone your pelvic muscles, the very center of you. Firm your abdominal muscles, alleviate lower back and urinary problems, and banish the bulge above your waist. Strengthen the muscles that affect your bladder, bowel, uterus, groin, and the walls of your vagina. Enhance your physical ability to enjoy sex.

Do the movements—Front, Center, Back, Center—to the beat of your music. Move as if you were hinged at the waist, keeping your upper body still.

When you are comfortable with your exercise and the music, skip the center stop and move your pelvis rhythmically forward and back. If your music slows, rotate your pelvis in a circle to the right and left.

1 EXOTIC, EROTIC PELVIC SHIFT

Tuck your buttocks under and push your pubic bone forward. Tip your pelvis back. Tighten all the muscles you can, inside and out.

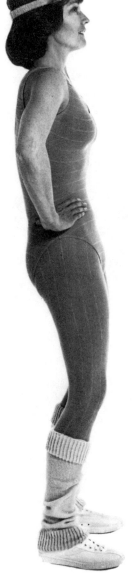

FRONT

The music should remind you of a Middle Eastern belly dancer, a West Indian entertainer.

Suggestions:

1. "Shame and Scandal," Alston Bair, *Live,* Federal
2. "Jamaica Farewell," Harry Belafonte, *Belafonte at Carnegie Hall,* RCA Victor
3. "Chattanooga Choo Choo," Ray Charles, *The Genius Hits the Road,* ABC Paramount

2 Shift your pelvis forward. Stop in the center of the shift, standing straight.

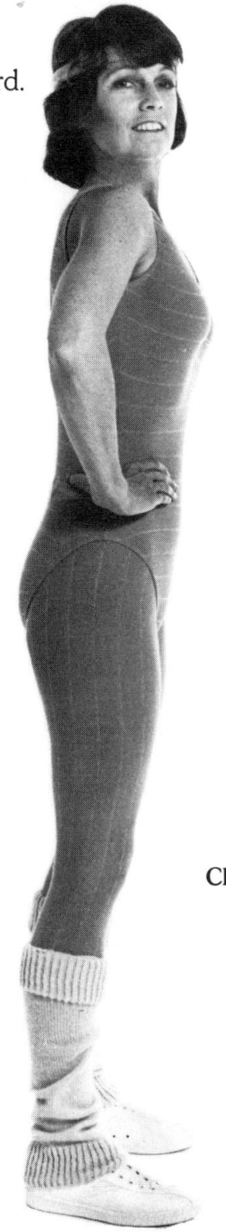

CENTER

3 Shift your buttocks out, relax your abdominal muscles, and gently arch your back.

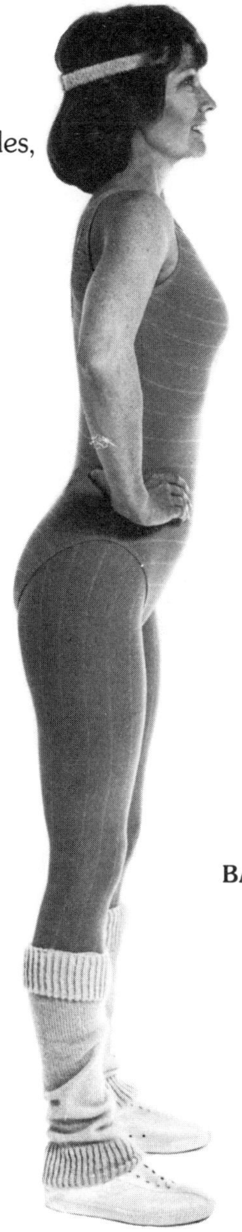

BACK

4 Shift your pelvis forward. Stop in the center.

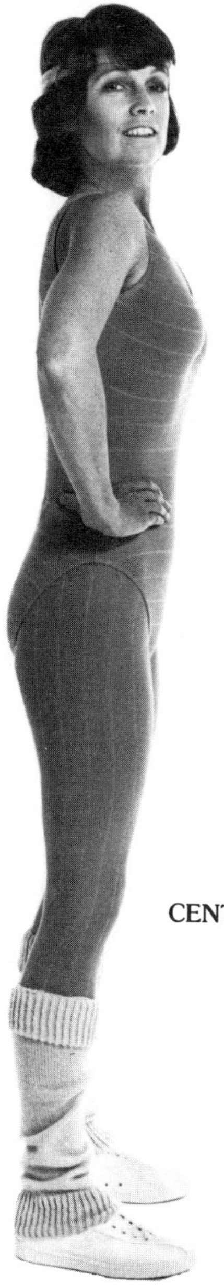

CENTER

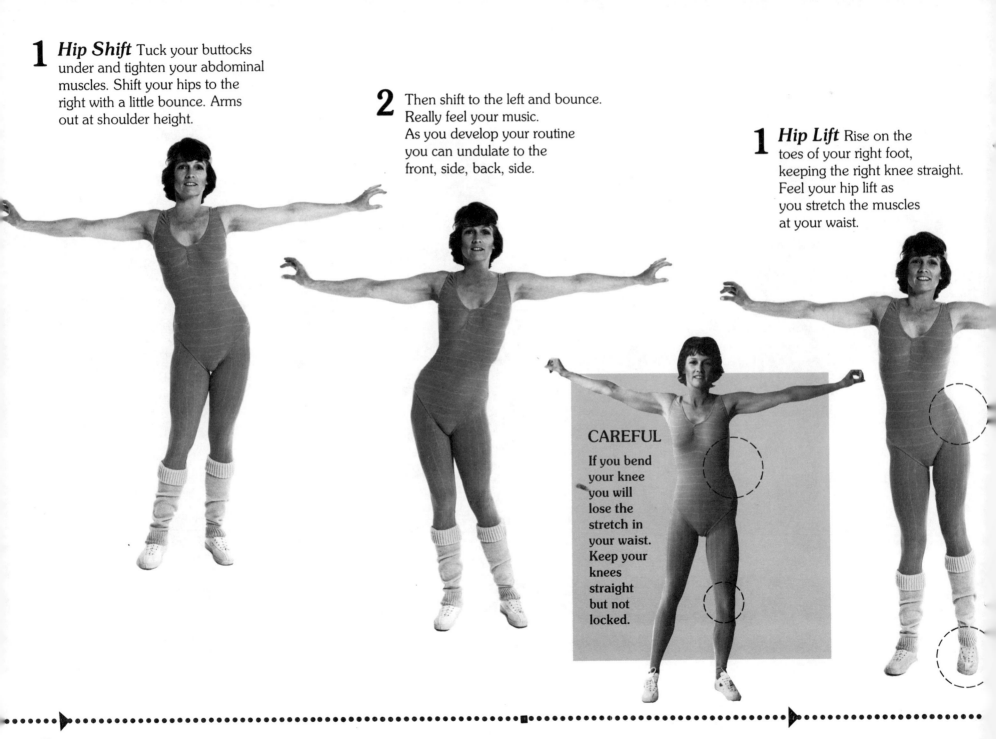

1 *Hip Shift* Tuck your buttocks under and tighten your abdominal muscles. Shift your hips to the right with a little bounce. Arms out at shoulder height.

2 Then shift to the left and bounce. Really feel your music. As you develop your routine you can undulate to the front, side, back, side.

1 *Hip Lift* Rise on the toes of your right foot, keeping the right knee straight. Feel your hip lift as you stretch the muscles at your waist.

CAREFUL
If you bend your knee you will lose the stretch in your waist. Keep your knees straight but not locked.

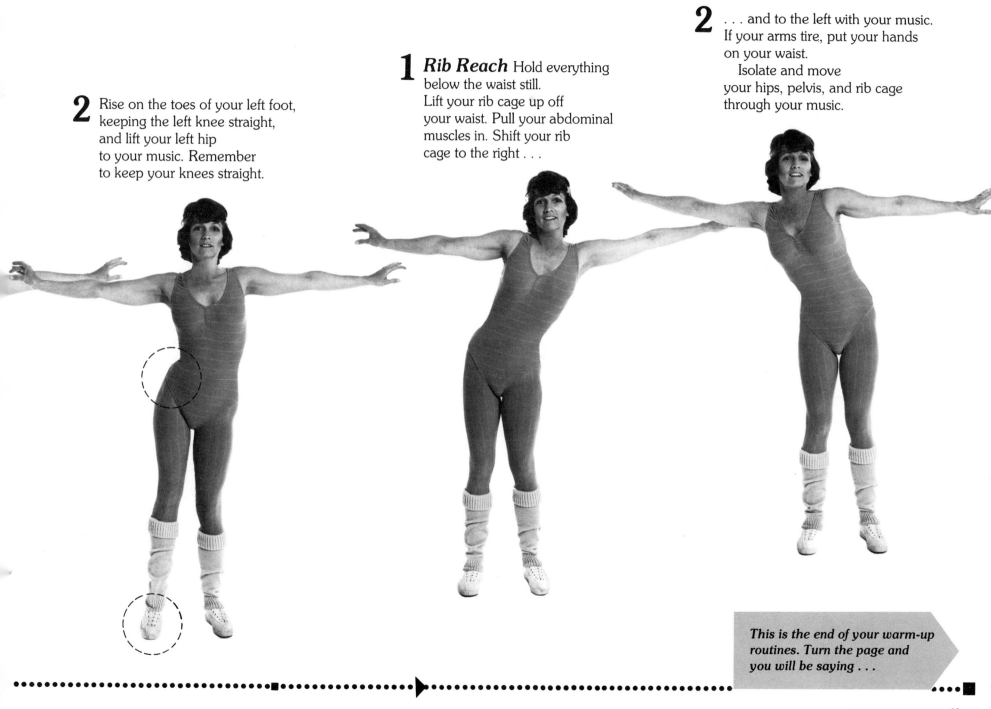

2 Rise on the toes of your left foot, keeping the left knee straight, and lift your left hip to your music. Remember to keep your knees straight.

1 *Rib Reach* Hold everything below the waist still. Lift your rib cage up off your waist. Pull your abdominal muscles in. Shift your rib cage to the right . . .

2 . . . and to the left with your music. If your arms tire, put your hands on your waist.
  Isolate and move your hips, pelvis, and rib cage through your music.

This is the end of your warm-up routines. Turn the page and you will be saying . . .

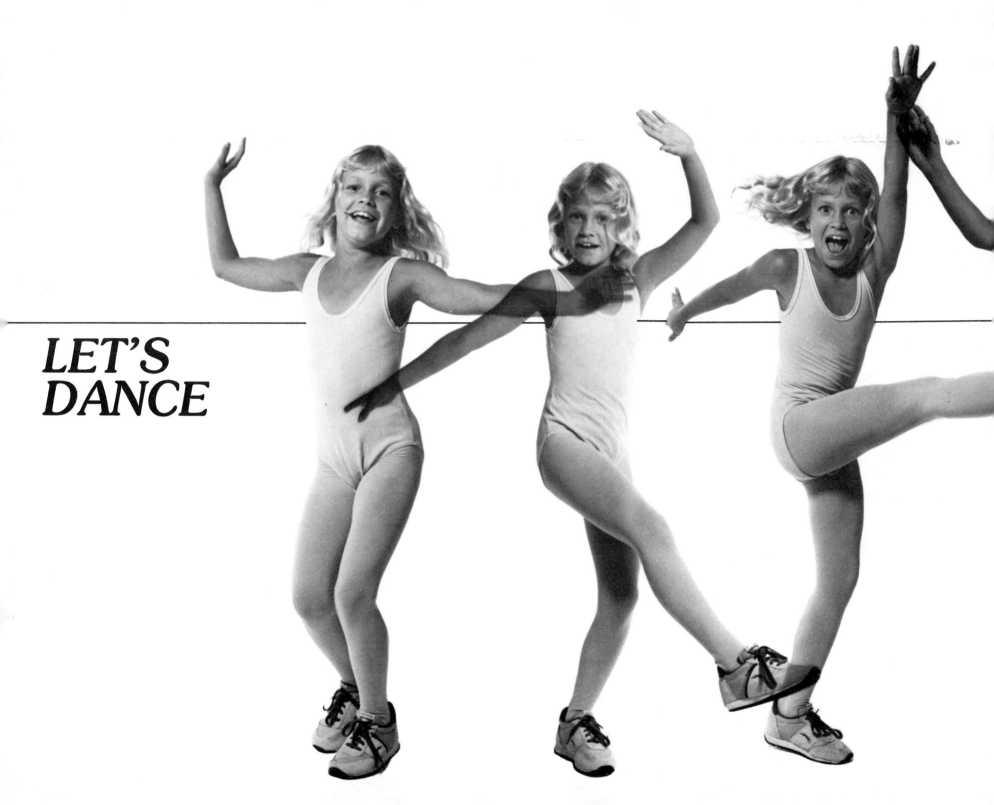

LET'S
DANCE

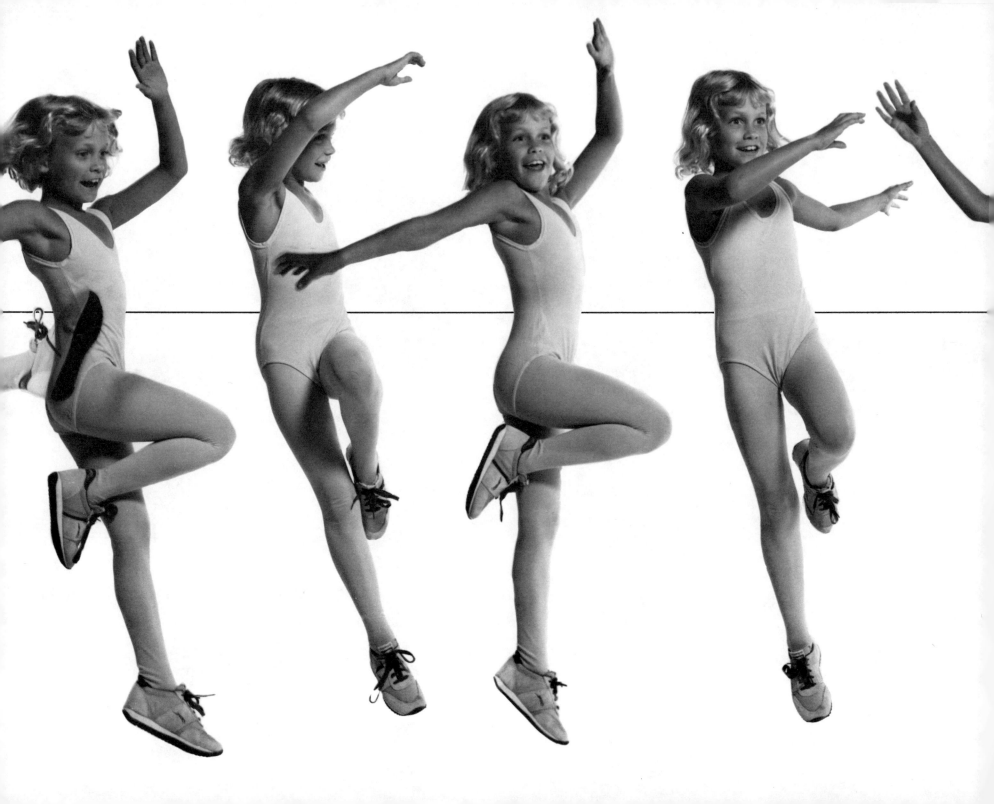

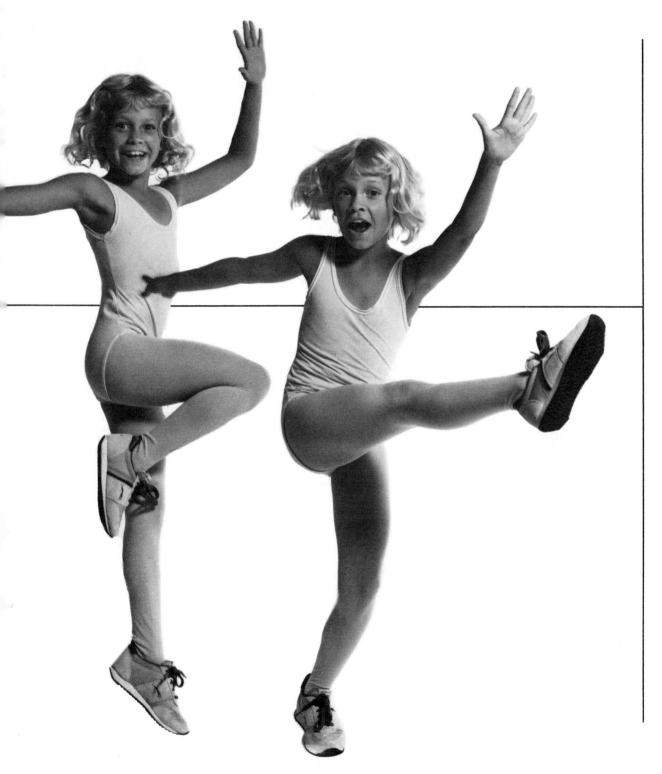

CONTENTS

*Dancing to a disco beat is a total body workout.
If you have carefully completed the warm-ups
on the previous pages, you are ready to dance.*

Doing the Disco

Never mind if you have never danced before. I designed this routine with you in mind. If you like disco music, follow me. You will stretch and warm your muscles from head to toe. You will begin to breathe deeply as you warm up your cardiovascular system. Listen to your music and hear the steady beat. Work your movements to that beat. Disco music is fun, but if you prefer, the dancing routine can be slowed way down and done to a rhythmic warm-up song. If you do that, disregard the bounce in the patterns, but enjoy the stretch in each exercise.

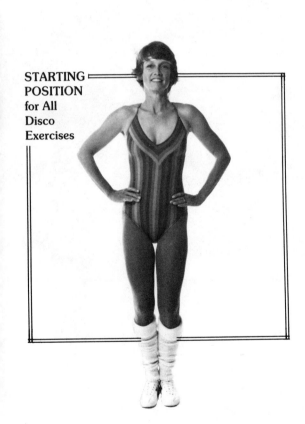

STARTING POSITION for All Disco Exercises

Stand tall, hands on hips, and listen to the beat. Get ready to move four steps to the right.

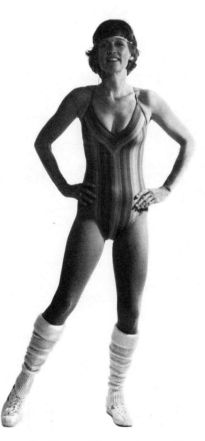

1 ***Step Together, Tap*** Step out on your right foot.

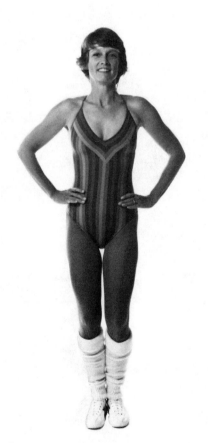

2 Bring your left foot to your right foot so that your feet are together.

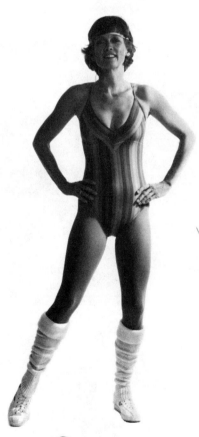

3 Step out on your right foot again.

The music
has a strong eight-count beat,
all strobe lights and glitter.
Suggestions:

1. "Fame," Irene Cara, *Fame,*
   RSO Records
2. "New York City Rhythm," Barry Manilow,
   Greatest Hits, Arista Records
3. "Dim All the Lights," Donna Summer,
   Bad Girl, Casablanca
   Records

Repeat Step Together, Tap to
the right and to the left until
you are comfortable and can
really feel your music.

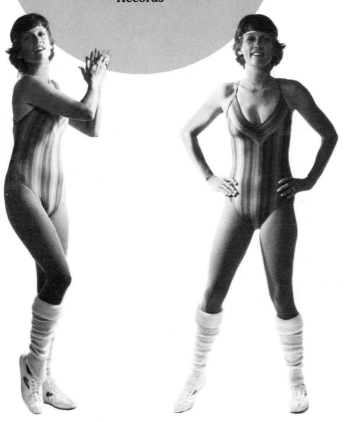
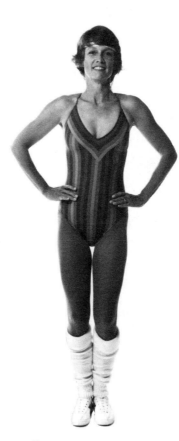
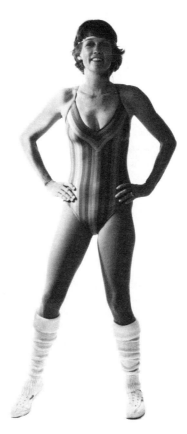
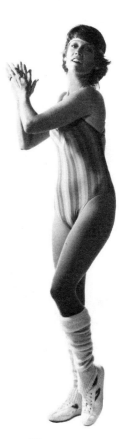

4 Tap your left toes just next
to your right foot and clap.

5 Now step out on
your left foot.

6 Step Together.

7 Step out on your
left foot again.

8 Tap and clap.

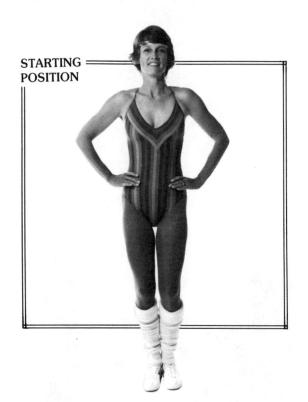

Stand tall, hands on hips.

ADVANCED
**Let's make the
Step Together, Tap
routine more aerobic.
Replace the tap
with a hop.**

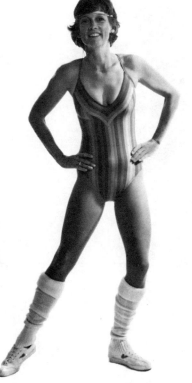

1 *STEP TOGETHER, HOP*
Step out on your right foot.

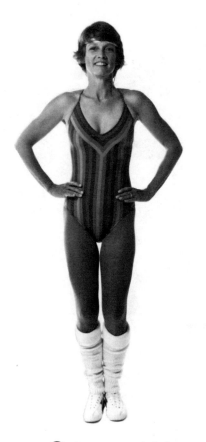

2 Bring your left foot
to your right foot.

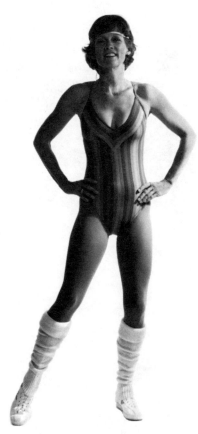

3 Step right . . .

ADVANCED

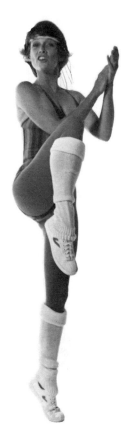 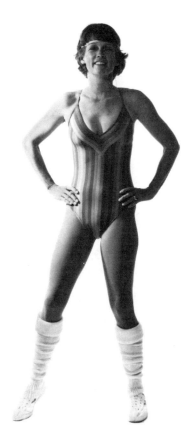 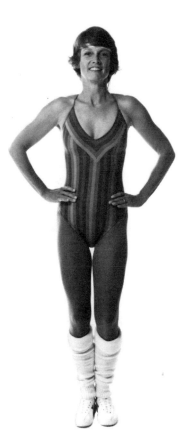 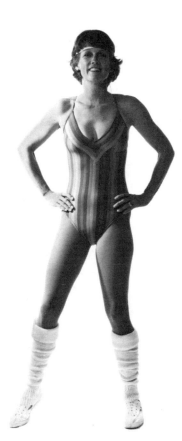 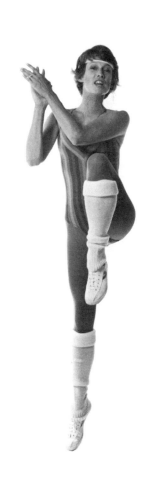

4 . . . and hop on your right foot, lifting your left knee as high as you can, and clap.

5 From your knee lift, step out on the left.

6 Bring your right foot in.

7 Step left . . .

8 . . . and hop on your left foot, and lift and clap!

ADVANCED

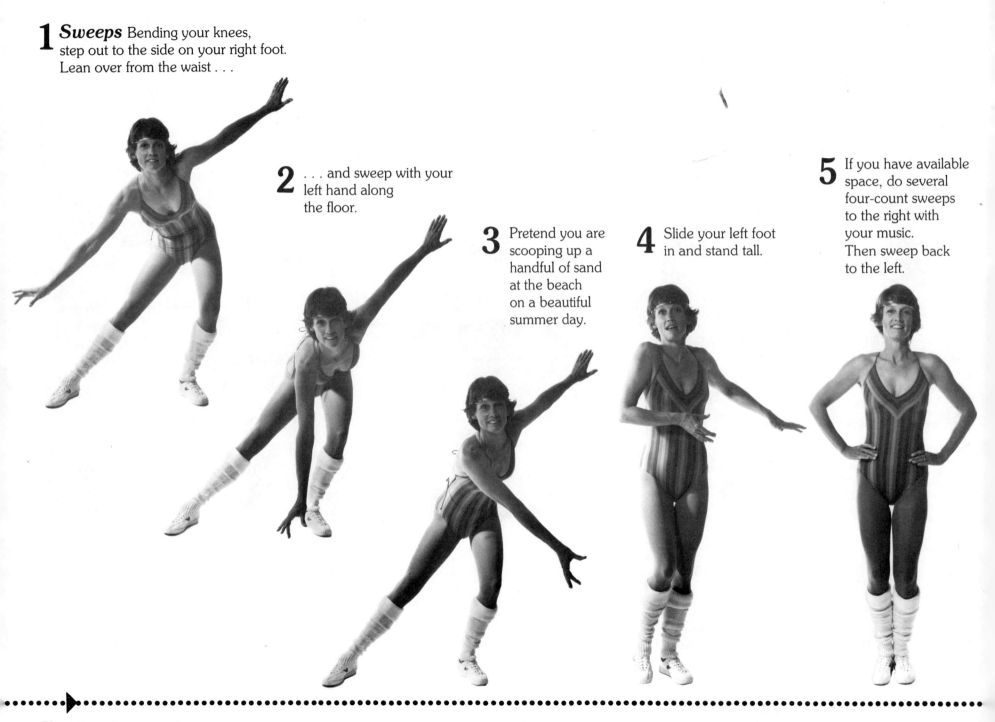

1 *Sweeps* Bending your knees, step out to the side on your right foot. Lean over from the waist . . .

2 . . . and sweep with your left hand along the floor.

3 Pretend you are scooping up a handful of sand at the beach on a beautiful summer day.

4 Slide your left foot in and stand tall.

5 If you have available space, do several four-count sweeps to the right with your music. Then sweep back to the left.

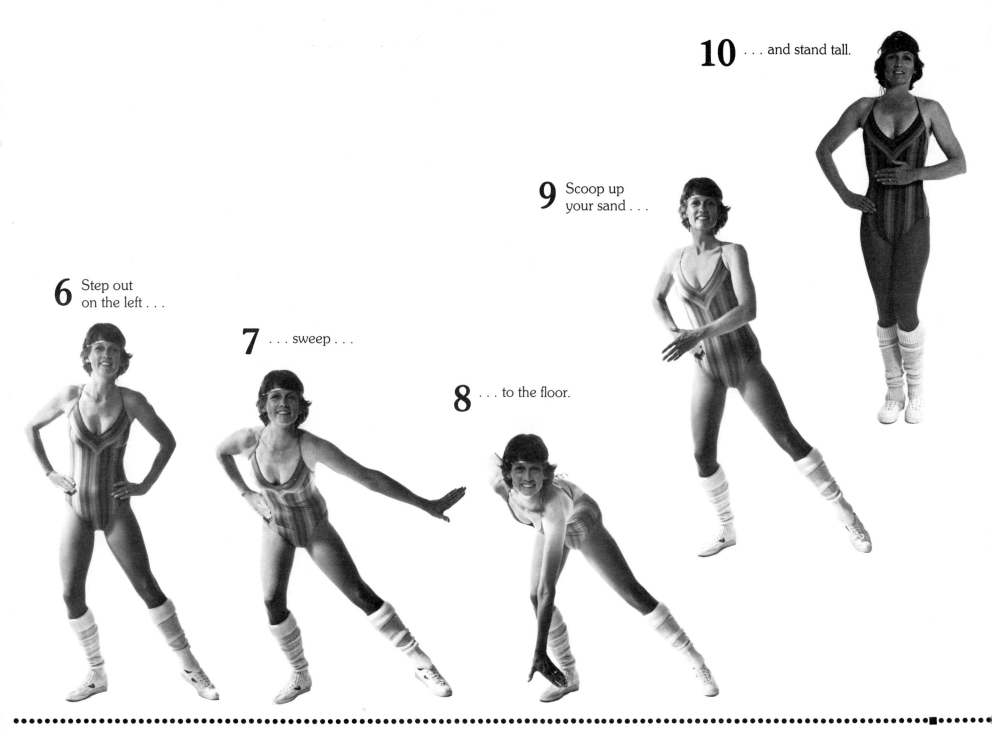

10 . . . and stand tall.

9 Scoop up
your sand . . .

6 Step out
on the left . . .

7 . . . sweep . . .

8 . . . to the floor.

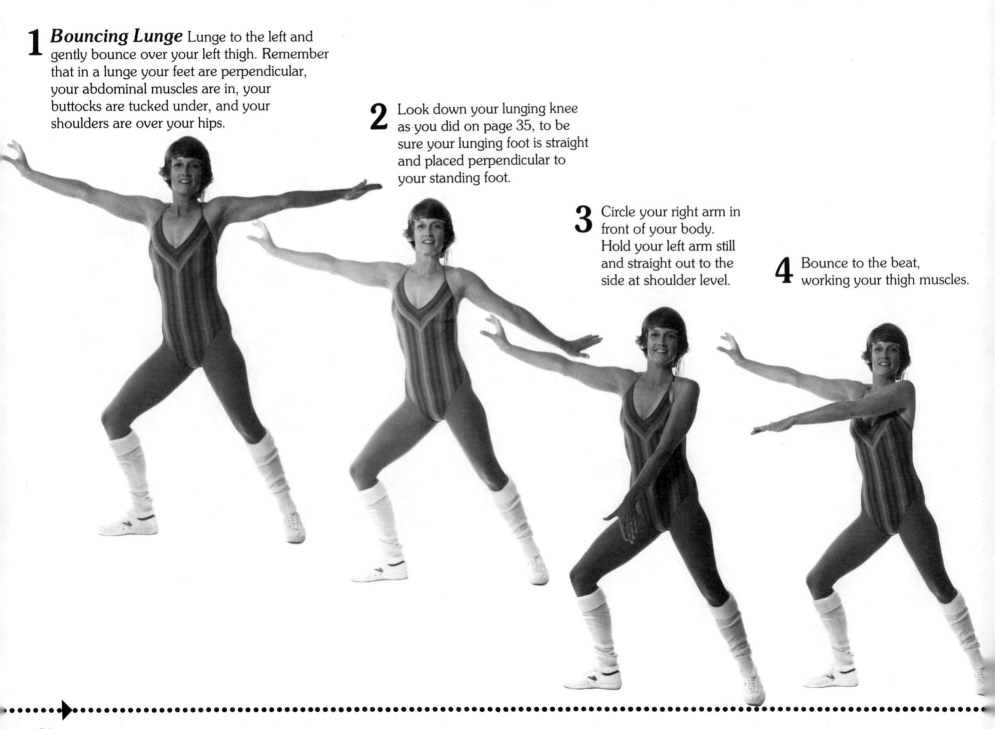

1 *Bouncing Lunge* Lunge to the left and gently bounce over your left thigh. Remember that in a lunge your feet are perpendicular, your abdominal muscles are in, your buttocks are tucked under, and your shoulders are over your hips.

2 Look down your lunging knee as you did on page 35, to be sure your lunging foot is straight and placed perpendicular to your standing foot.

3 Circle your right arm in front of your body. Hold your left arm still and straight out to the side at shoulder level.

4 Bounce to the beat, working your thigh muscles.

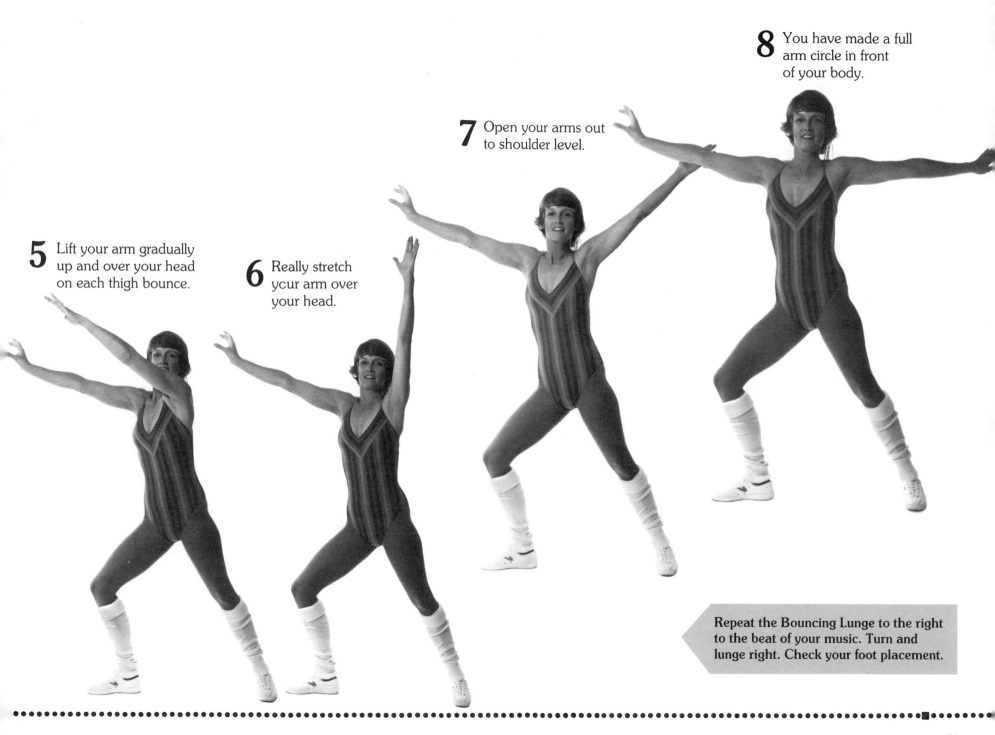

5 Lift your arm gradually up and over your head on each thigh bounce.

6 Really stretch ycur arm over your head.

7 Open your arms out to shoulder level.

8 You have made a full arm circle in front of your body.

Repeat the Bouncing Lunge to the right to the beat of your music. Turn and lunge right. Check your foot placement.

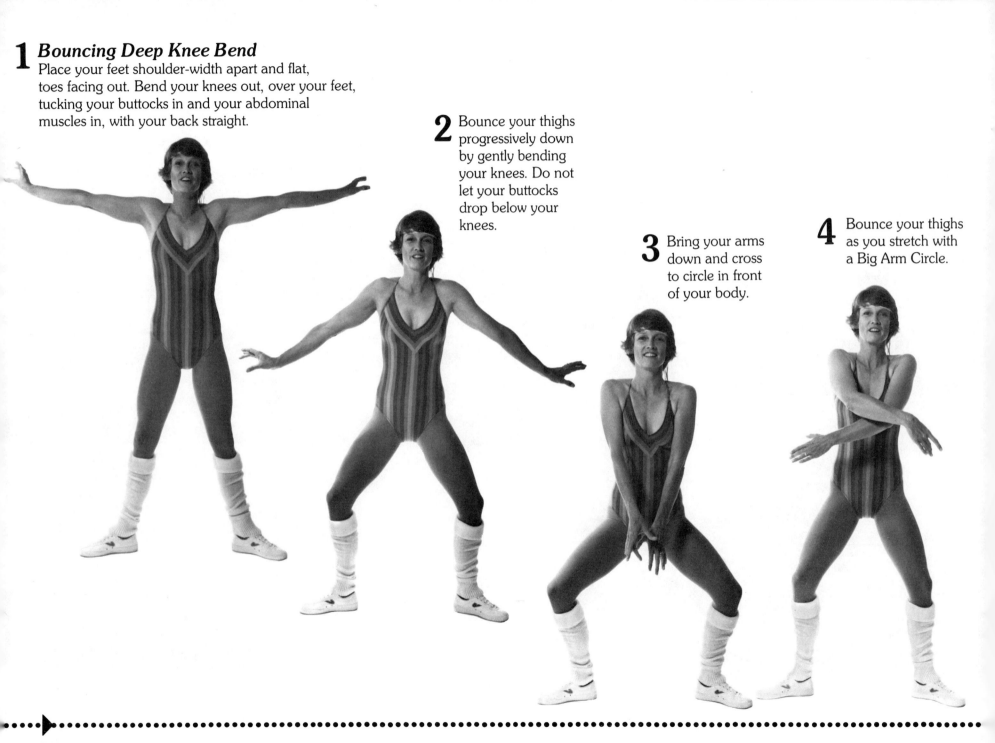

1 Bouncing Deep Knee Bend
Place your feet shoulder-width apart and flat, toes facing out. Bend your knees out, over your feet, tucking your buttocks in and your abdominal muscles in, with your back straight.

2 Bounce your thighs progressively down by gently bending your knees. Do not let your buttocks drop below your knees.

3 Bring your arms down and cross to circle in front of your body.

4 Bounce your thighs as you stretch with a Big Arm Circle.

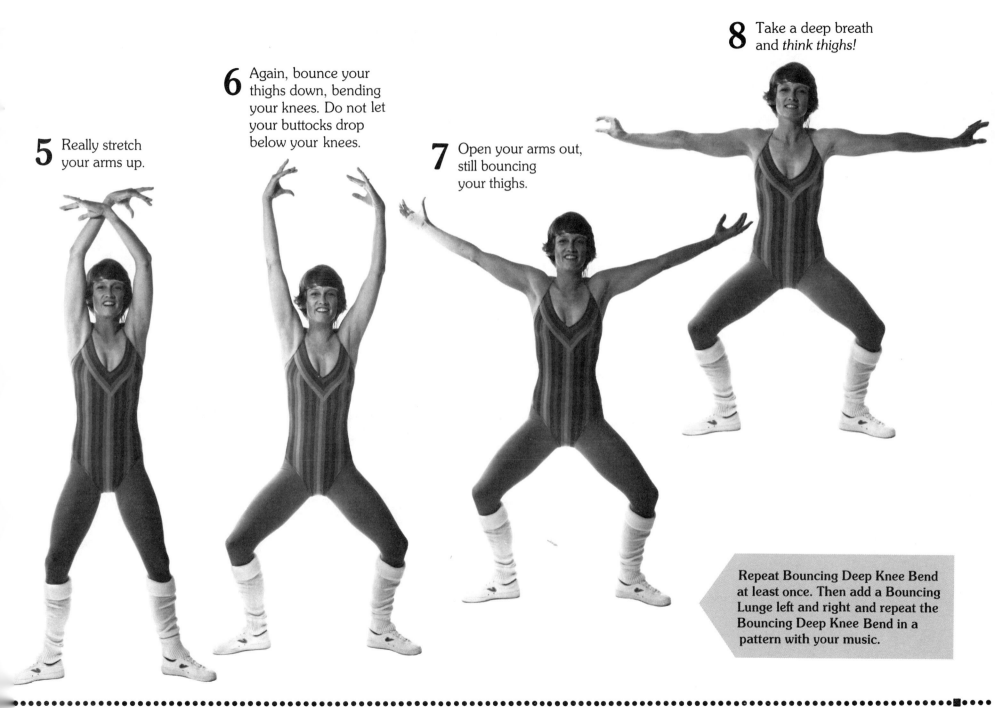

5 Really stretch your arms up.

6 Again, bounce your thighs down, bending your knees. Do not let your buttocks drop below your knees.

7 Open your arms out, still bouncing your thighs.

8 Take a deep breath and *think thighs!*

Repeat Bouncing Deep Knee Bend at least once. Then add a Bouncing Lunge left and right and repeat the Bouncing Deep Knee Bend in a pattern with your music.

1 **Working Your Feet In**
Place your feet apart and your toes out. Hands on your hips.By keeping your heels down during this pattern you are working your lower leg muscles.

2 Pivot on your heels so that your toes face front, and gently bounce your knees twice, keeping your heels down. Feel the stretch in the back of your legs.

3 Pivot on the balls of your feet so that your heels are in and your toes out, and bounce twice.

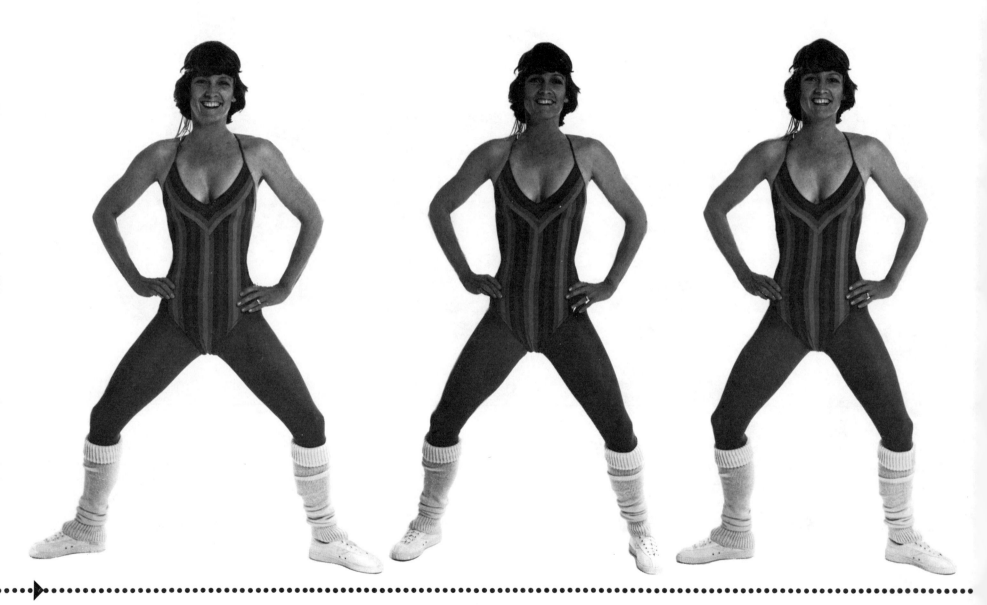

4 Pivot on your heels so that your toes face front, and bounce twice. The space between your feet is getting smaller.

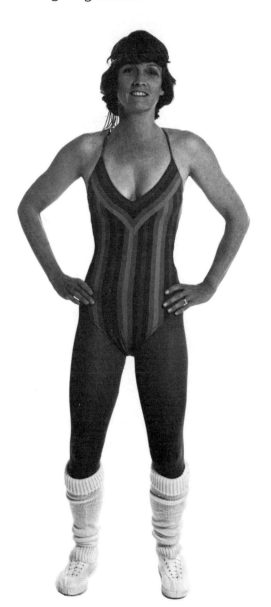

5 Pivot on the balls of your feet so that your heels are in, and bounce twice.

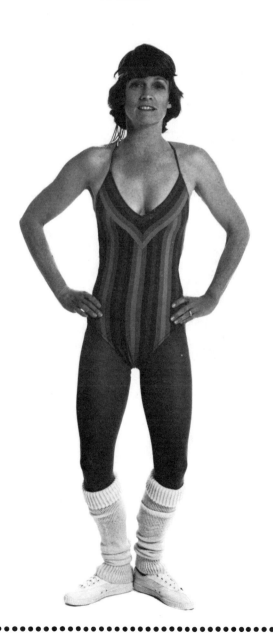

6 Pivot on your heels so that your toes are together, and bounce twice. You've run out of space! Go directly into the next pattern.

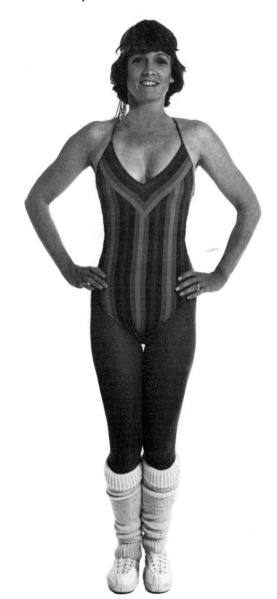

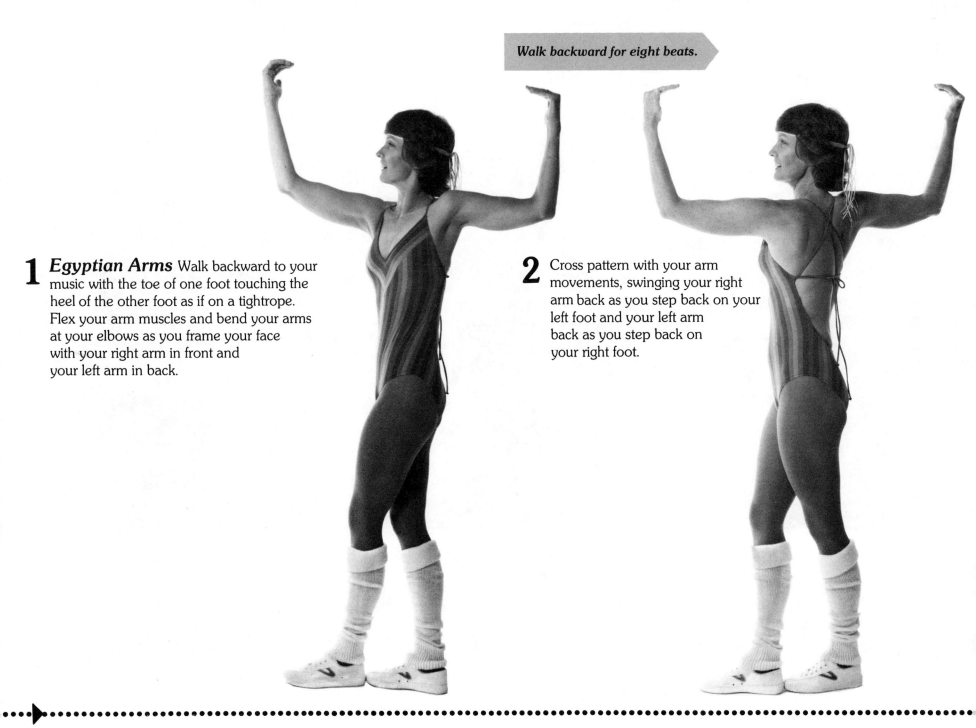

Walk backward for eight beats.

1 *Egyptian Arms* Walk backward to your music with the toe of one foot touching the heel of the other foot as if on a tightrope. Flex your arm muscles and bend your arms at your elbows as you frame your face with your right arm in front and your left arm in back.

2 Cross pattern with your arm movements, swinging your right arm back as you step back on your left foot and your left arm back as you step back on your right foot.

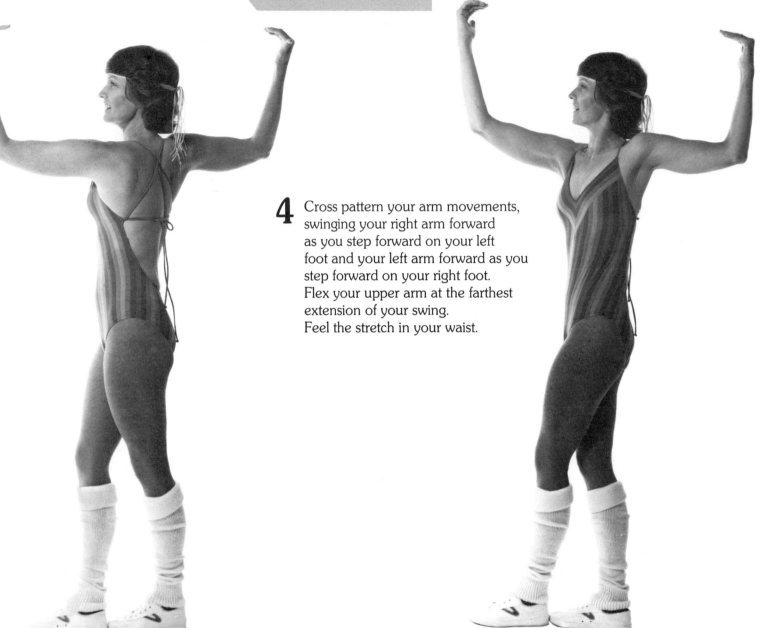

Keep your arms at shoulder level as you exercise your waist, chest, and arm muscles. Keep your hips forward and swing at the waist. THINK SPHINX.

3 Walk forward now, heel to toe. Stay on an imaginary tightrope.

4 Cross pattern your arm movements, swinging your right arm forward as you step forward on your left foot and your left arm forward as you step forward on your right foot. Flex your upper arm at the farthest extension of your swing. Feel the stretch in your waist.

After your last swing on your Egyptian Arms pattern, stand in place, ready for Push-Pull.

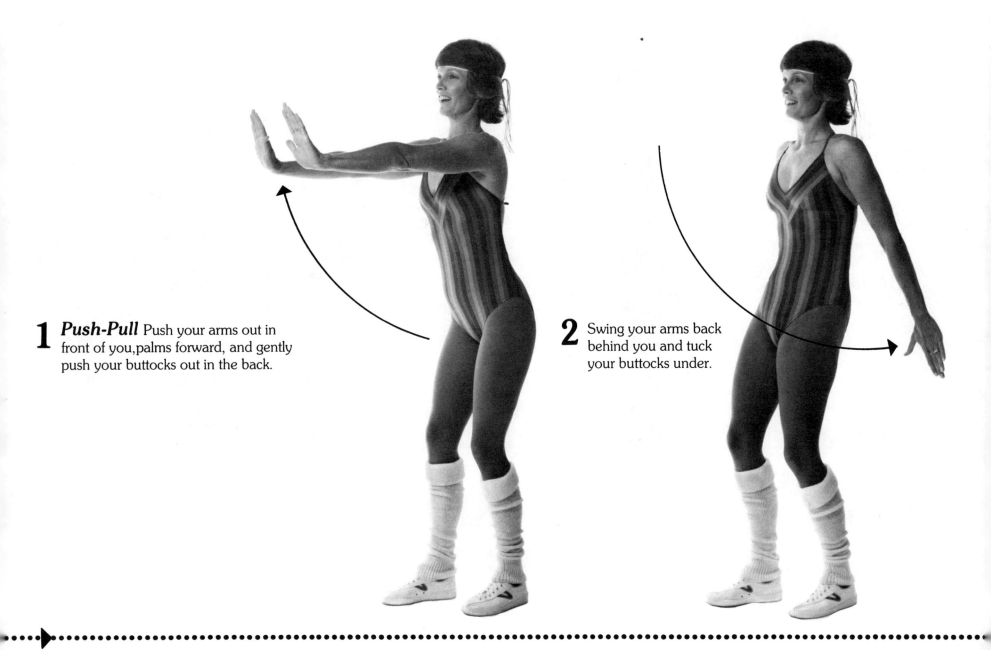

1 ***Push-Pull*** Push your arms out in front of you, palms forward, and gently push your buttocks out in the back.

2 Swing your arms back behind you and tuck your buttocks under.

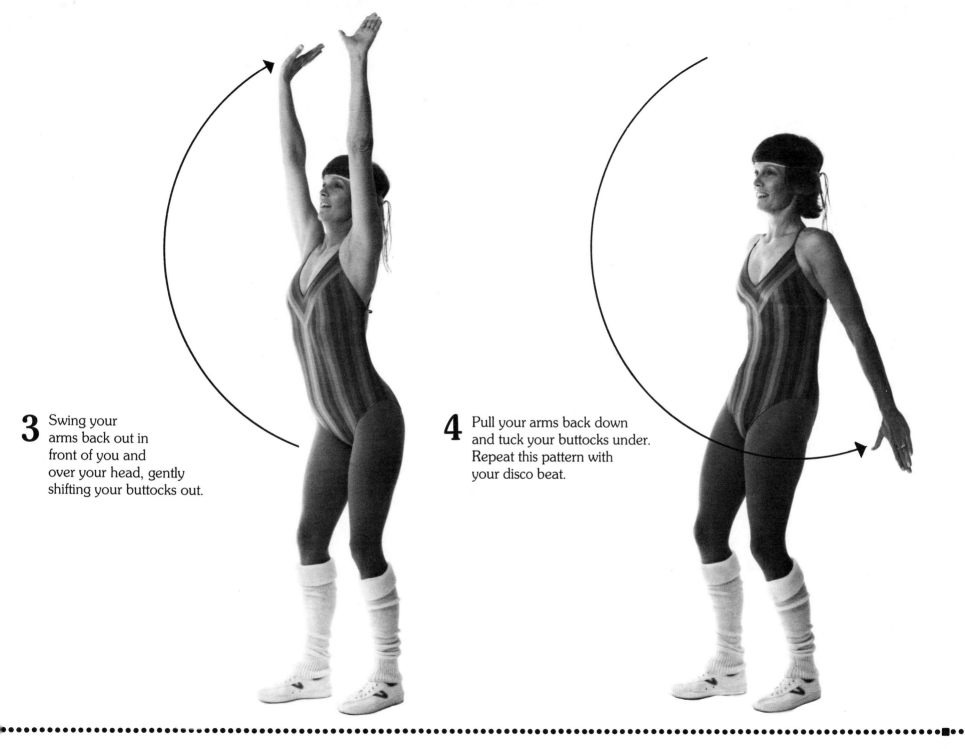

3 Swing your arms back out in front of you and over your head, gently shifting your buttocks out.

4 Pull your arms back down and tuck your buttocks under. Repeat this pattern with your disco beat.

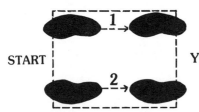

START

You are painting a square on the floor
with your feet.

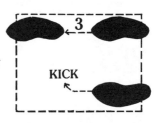

KICK

Place your feet shoulder-width
apart, toes to the front,
knees relaxed.

1 **The Square**
Step straight back
with your right foot . . .

2 . . . then back with your
left foot, so that your
feet are shoulder-
width apart again.

3 Step forward on
your right foot.

4 Kick your left
leg up and clap.

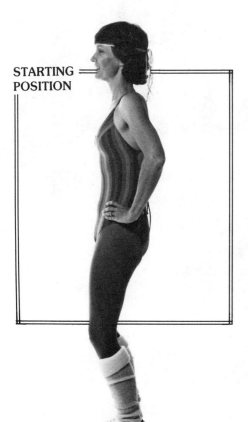

**STARTING
POSITION**

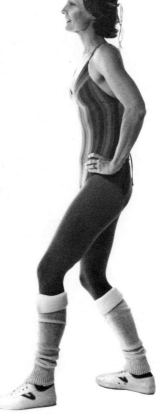

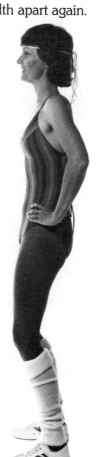

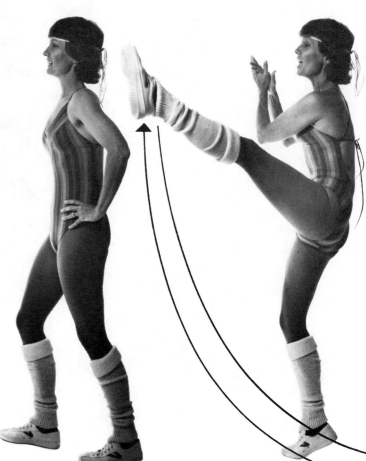

You've got the feel of it now!
Repeat your square as many times
as you like with your music.

5 From your kick,
step straight back
with your left foot . . .

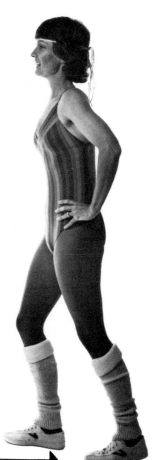

6 . . . then back with your
right foot so that your
feet are shoulder-width
apart again.

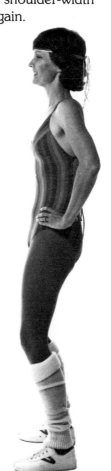

7 Step forward on your left foot . . .

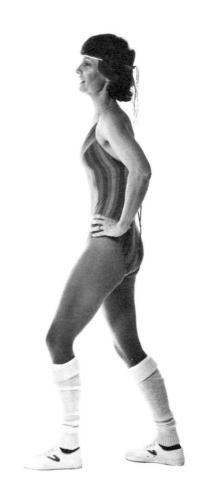

8 . . . and kick your right leg and clap.
Really lift your leg with your
thigh muscle, and keep your
standing foot flat.

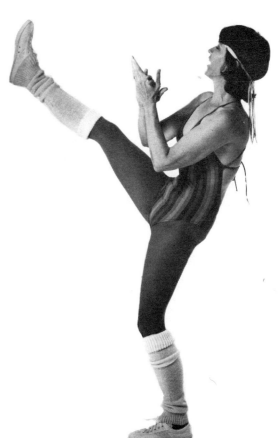

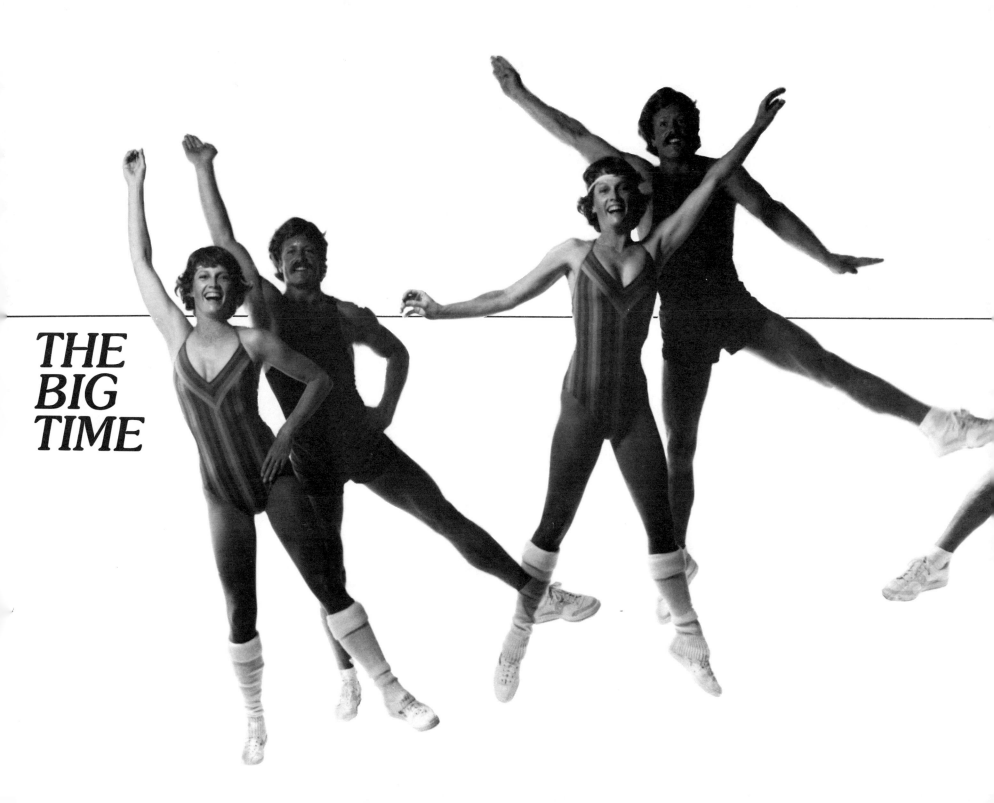

THE
BIG
TIME

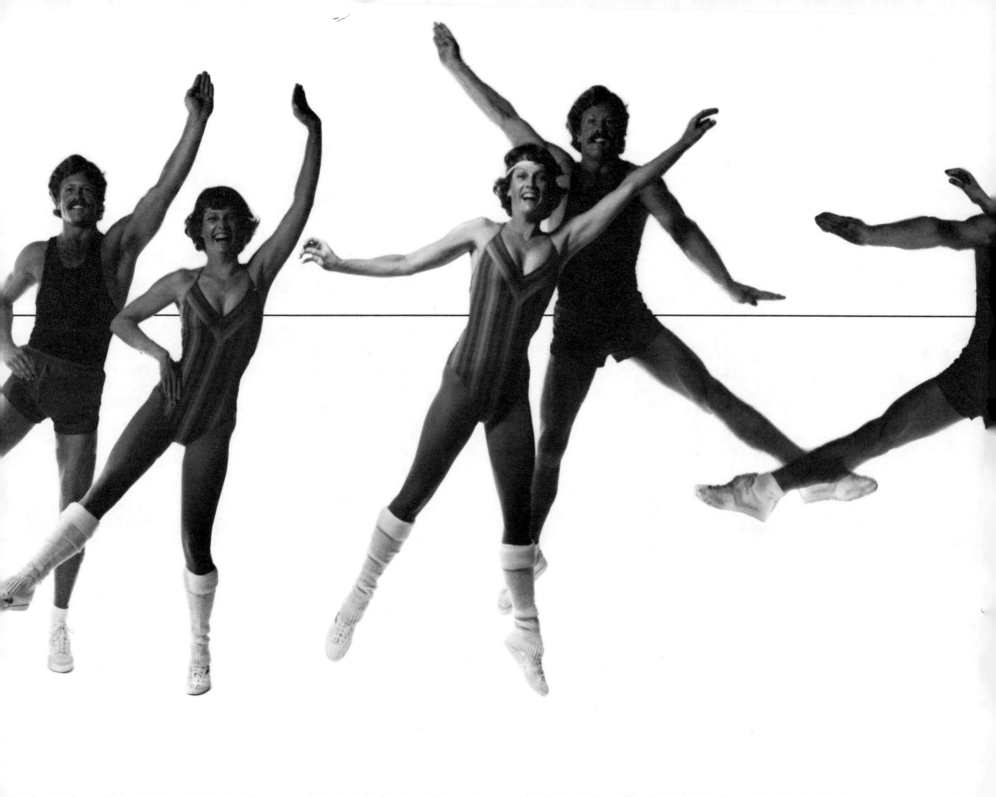

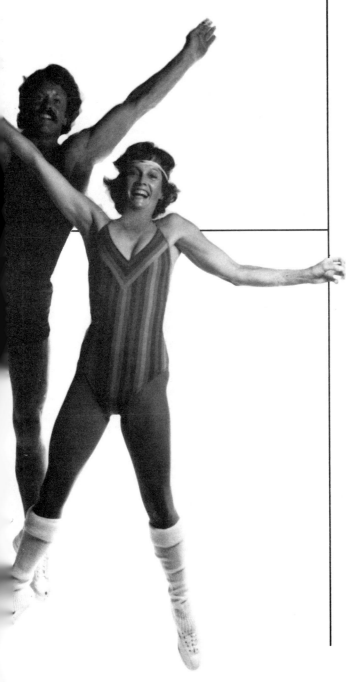

CONTENTS

* Exercises marked with an asterisk are the only ones that change in each pattern. Notice how the other exercises repeat themselves.

You've made it to The Big Time! Get ready to enjoy wonderful new energy as you exercise your total body, inside and out, strengthen your heart and lungs, and burn up unwanted calories.
    The Big Time consists of three aerobic conditioning routines that I call Aerobic Highs.

Each Aerobic High is made up of three patterns —Acceleration, Exhilaration, and Jubilation— and each of these patterns consists of three exercises. So before you tackle The Big Time, read through the entire section and familiarize yourself with the patterns. Especially note when to measure your pulse. It's time to get "really aerobic."

When you turn on your music, commit yourself to exercise until the music ends. If you forget the aerobic patterns, jog in place. If you tire, walk in place, keeping the beat of the music, and continue with the patterns when you feel rested. What's important is to keep moving until the music ends. Whether you are walking, jogging, or following the patterns exactly, or creating a combination of moves that feel even better to you, keep going. You can do it!
    You can adjust the aerobic level of each routine by adjusting the height of your jog. The higher you lift your knees, the more strenuous the routine becomes. Inversely, jogging with lowered knees or walking in place will help you "rest" while you maintain your aerobic momentum. Do what's comfortable for you.
    You should experience some breathlessness, but not be completely winded. If you can sing with your music or carry on a conversation while exercising, the aerobic pace is right for you. The music itself should give you a burst of energy and help you sprint to the finish.

Aerobic High I
ACCELERATION

Fit this pattern to your music's phrases. How long
you work through it is up to you. Do what feels
good, but try to fit it into one minute. Then go on
to the next patterns—Exhilaration and Jubilation. If
you finish Jubilation before your music ends, start
again with Acceleration. When the music ends
(about three minutes), be ready to take your pulse.

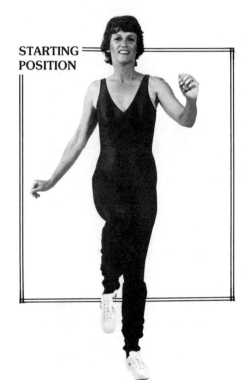

STARTING
POSITION

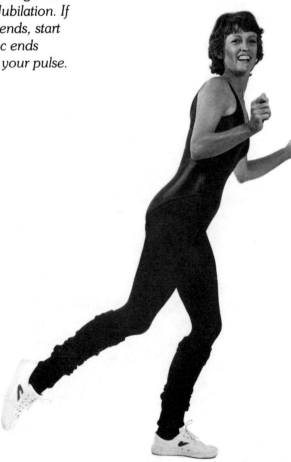

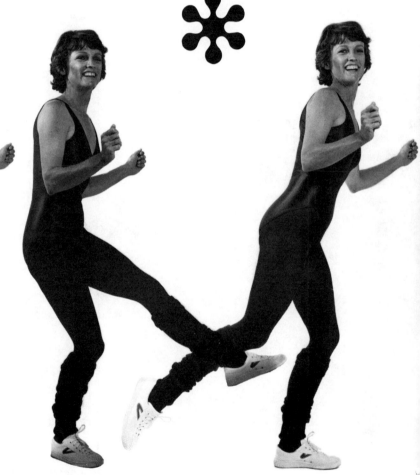

Jog in place. Lift your knees up.
When you land, use as much of your foot
as you can, rolling from your heel
to the ball of your foot.

1 *Rock 2-3, Kick*
Rock forward on
your left foot . . .

2 . . . rock back on
your right foot . . .

3 . . . rock forward on
your left foot . . .

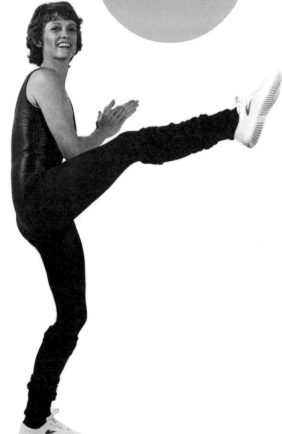

Suggestion:
"Jump Shout Boogie,"
Barry Manilow,
Greatest Hits,
Arista Records

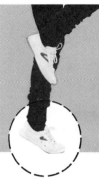

CAREFUL
Adjust your patterns to your space. Use as much room as you have available. Tighten your pelvic area while you are doing the aerobic patterns, in order to exercise the pelvic muscles so essential for bladder control and abdominal strength. Avoid jogging on your toes. This may cause painful shins and lower back discomfort.

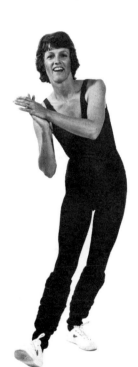

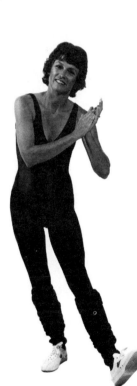

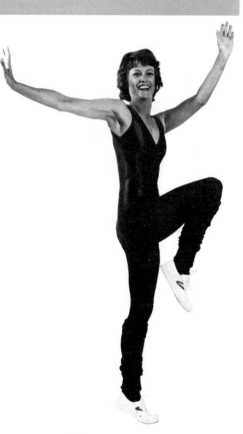

4 . . . and kick your right leg up, lifting with your thigh muscle and keeping your standing foot flat. Clap your hands with your kick. For a detailed review of Rock 2-3, Kick, see page 48.

1 *Peppy Pull Back* Step back on your right leg. By bending your right knee but keeping the heel down you will "sit" back over your right foot. Keeping your left leg straight, flex your left foot, toes up. Clap! Step back on your left leg . . .

2 . . . and "sit" over your left foot, flexing your right foot. Clap! Pull back as far as your space allows.

Skip Skip forward, cross patterning; lift your right knee as your left arm swings forward, and lift your left knee as your right arm swings forward.

Aerobic High I
EXHILARATION

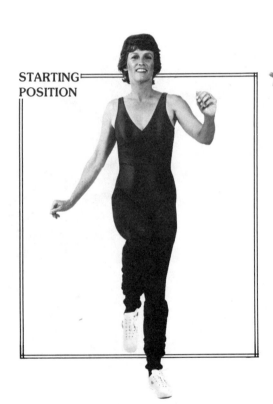

STARTING POSITION

Jog in place.
Remember, if you should tire,
walk in place.

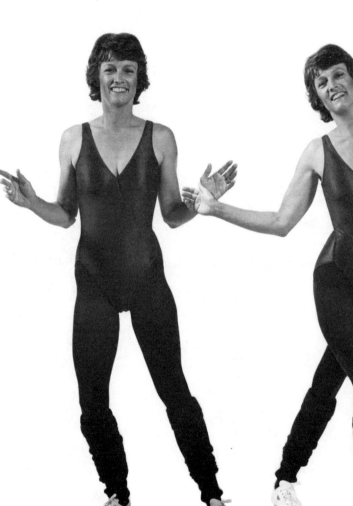

1 *Sunflower*
Step out to the side
on your right foot.

2 Cross over in the
front with your
left foot.

3 Step out on your
right foot again.

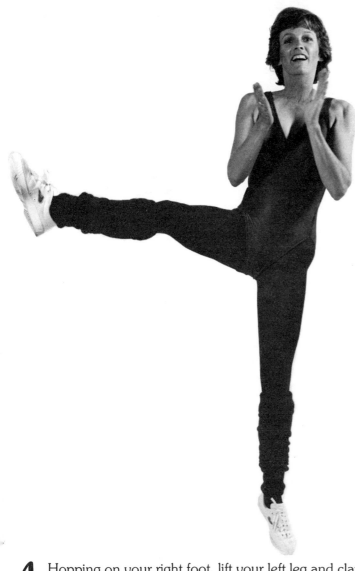

Repeat until you are comfortable with the pattern and with your music. For a detailed review of the Sunflower, see pages 50–51.

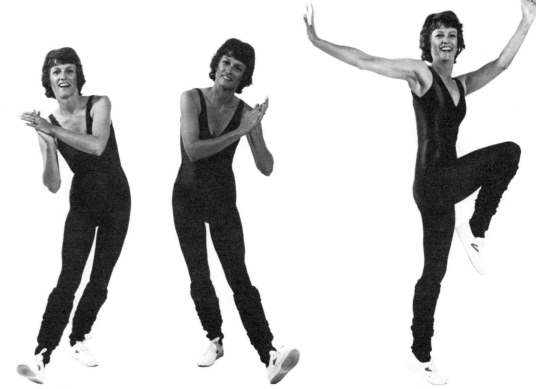

4 Hopping on your right foot, lift your left leg and clap. Step out on your left leg and Sunflower back in the other direction. Cross over in the front with your right foot, step on your left foot again, and lift your right leg and clap, hopping on your left foot.

1 *Peppy Pull Back* Step back on your right leg. "Sit" back over your right foot. As you flex your left foot, feel the stretch along the back of your left leg . . .

2 . . . and along the back of your right leg.

Skip Really swing your arms.

Aerobic High I
JUBILATION

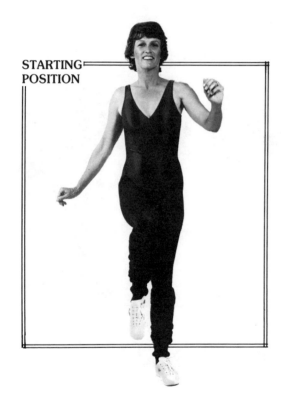

STARTING
POSITION

Jog in place.
Knees up in front of you.

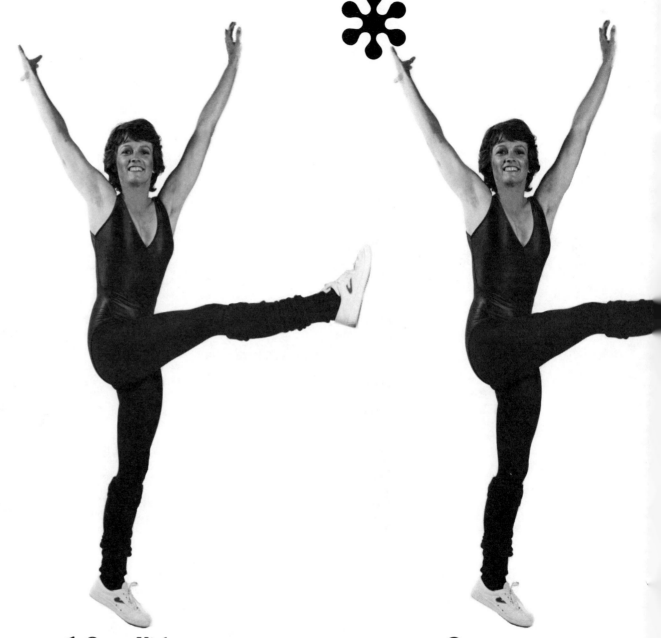

1 *Cross Kick* Lift your leg with your thigh muscle, kicking across your body. Keep your knee straight and point your toes. Your standing foot is flat.

2 Kick with the other leg. For a detailed review of Cross Kick, see page 49.

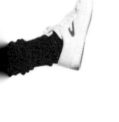

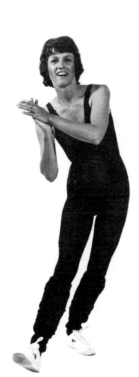

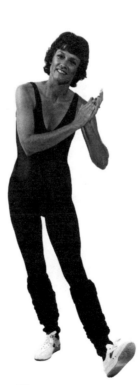

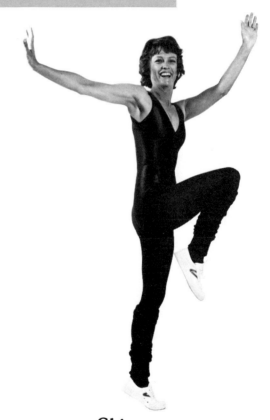

1 *Peppy Pull Back*
Step back on your right leg, sit, flex your foot.

2 Step back on your left leg . . . and stretch.

Skip
Lift your knees.

Aerobic High II
ACCELERATION

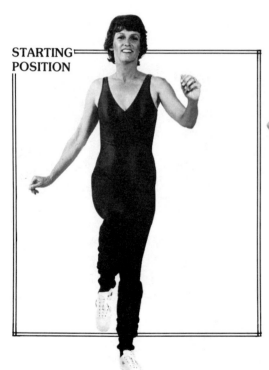

STARTING POSITION

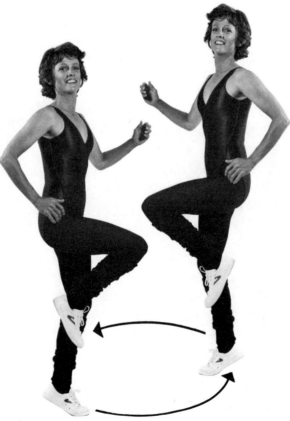

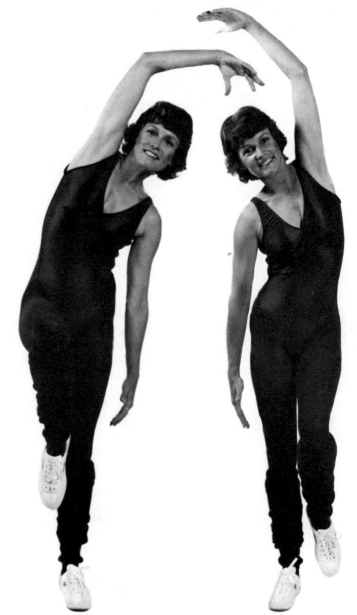

Jog in place. Knees up in front. Don't forget to breathe. Remember to land as full-footed as possible.

1 ***Jog Around Yourself*** Knees up in front.

2 Jog around yourself in a circle to the right and in a circle to the left.

1 ***Jump and Side Lean 2-3*** Leaning to the right, jump to the side onto the right foot. Holding your lean, shift to the left foot, then shift to the right. Repeat Jump and Side Lean 2-3 to the left.

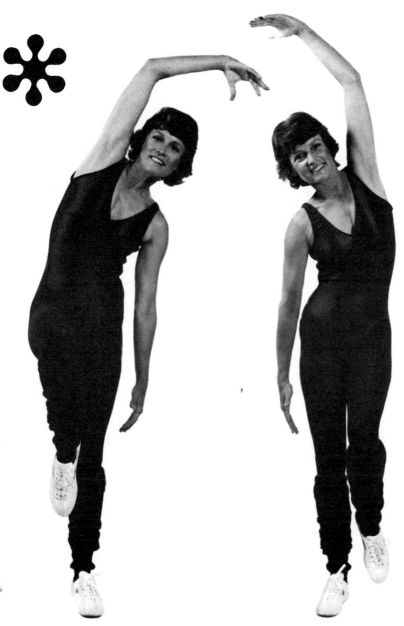

Music Suggestion:

"Love's Been a Little Bit Hard on Me," Juice Newton, *Quiet Lies*, Capitol Records

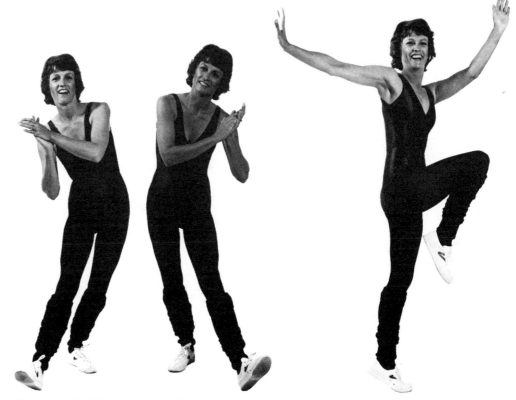

2 Repeat Jump and Side Lean 2-3 to the right and to the left.

1 *Peppy Pull Back* Step back on your right leg. Clap.

2 Step back on your left leg. Clap.

Skip Really swing out.

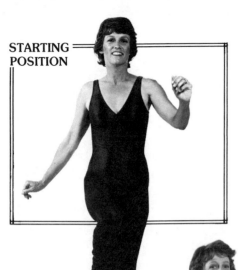

Aerobic High II
EXHILARATION

Jog in place.

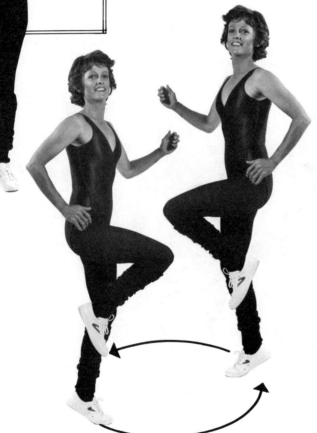

1 *Jog Around Yourself* Jog in a small circle around yourself to the right . . .

2 . . . and to the left.

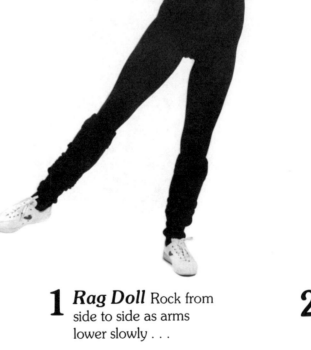

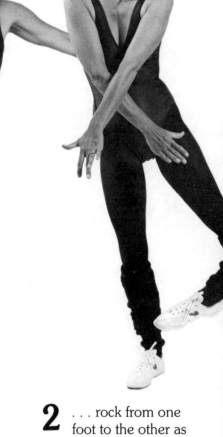

1 *Rag Doll* Rock from side to side as arms lower slowly . . .

2 . . . rock from one foot to the other as arms cross in front . . .

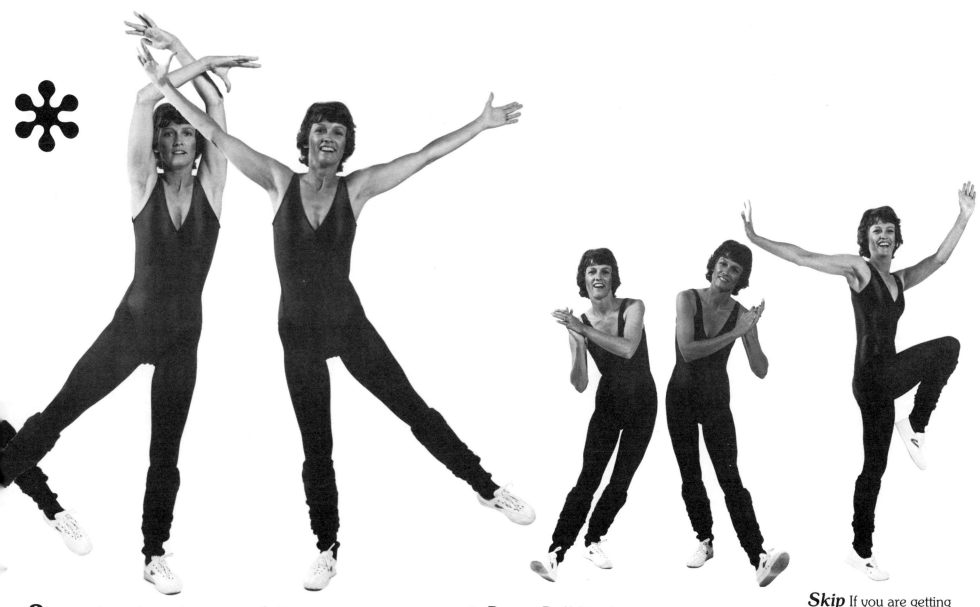

3 . . . and complete with a Big Arm Circle, still rocking side to side.

4 Repeat to your music and feel like a bouncy rag doll.

1 *Peppy Pull Back* Step back on your right leg. Stretch and clap.

2 Step back on your left leg. Clap.

Skip If you are getting breathless, walk in place, but if you feel *full of energy*, really lift your knees and swing your arms as you skip.

Aerobic High II
JUBILATION

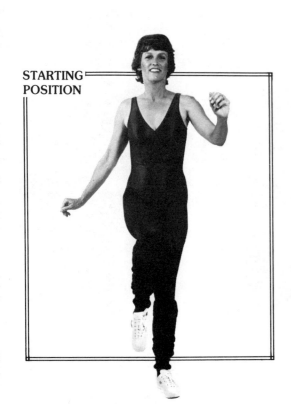

STARTING
POSITION

Jog in place.
Knees up and exhale.

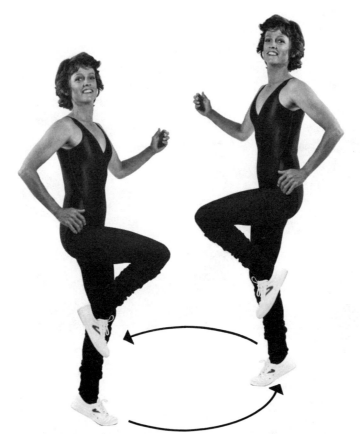

1 *Jog Around Yourself*
Smile, you can do it.
Lift your knees.

2 Take deep
breaths.

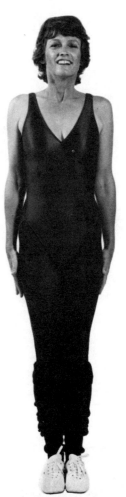

1 *Jumping Jacks*
Feet together and
arms at your sides.

2

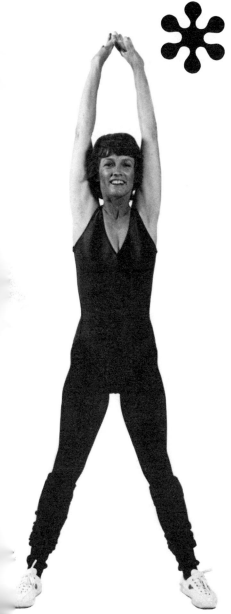

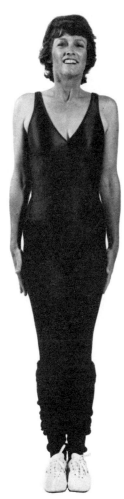

If you finish this routine before your music ends, just repeat the patterns until it does.

CAREFUL
When your music ends, count your active pulse for six seconds. If your active pulse is below, at, or only ten above your guideline, and if you feel good, you can move right on to Aerobic High III. If your active pulse is more than ten above your guideline, take a brisk walk around your exercise space, have a drink of water, and go on to the slimnastics.

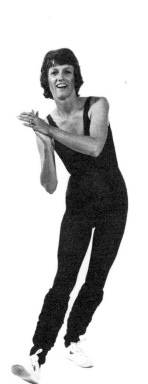

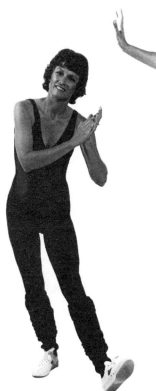

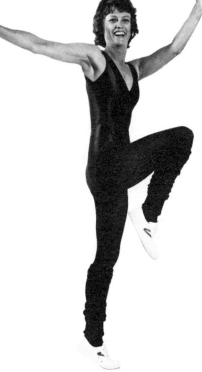

Hold your pelvic and abdominal muscles in as you jump feet apart and clap overhead.

3 Jump and put your feet together and hands to your sides.

1 *Peppy Pull Back*
Sit back on your right and stretch.

2 Sit back on your left and stretch.

Skip
Lift your knees.

Aerobic High III
ACCELERATION

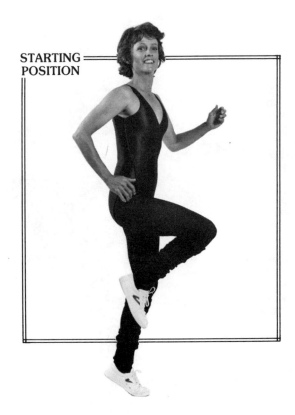

STARTING
POSITION

Jog in place. *Think thin.*

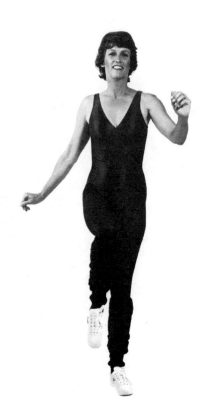

Jog Forward and Backward
Jog forward into your space. Without turning, jog backward. Knees up.

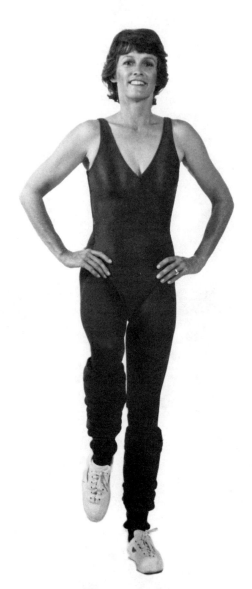

1 Tighten and Hop Pull your buttocks tightly together. Jump on the right foot four times.

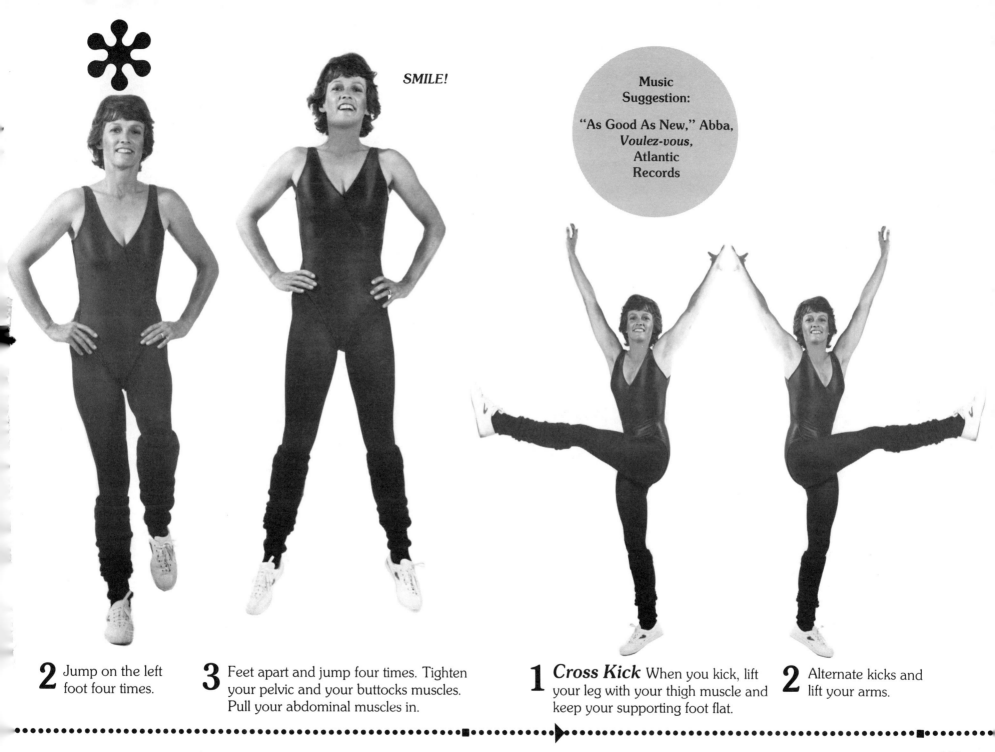

SMILE!

2 Jump on the left foot four times.

3 Feet apart and jump four times. Tighten your pelvic and your buttocks muscles. Pull your abdominal muscles in.

1 *Cross Kick* When you kick, lift your leg with your thigh muscle and keep your supporting foot flat.

2 Alternate kicks and lift your arms.

Aerobic High III
EXHILARATION

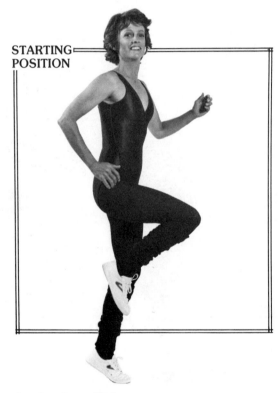

STARTING
POSITION

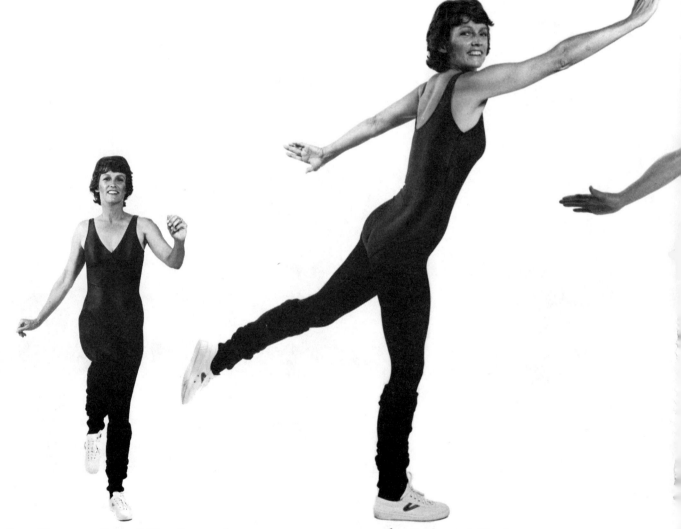

Jog in place. Relax your arms.

Jog Forward and Backward Jog forward into your space. Without turning around, jog backward. As you jog backward, feel the stretch in the back of your legs. Marathon runners, during a long training period, sometimes run a mile or so backward to reverse the stress on their leg muscles.

1 ***Jog and Swing*** Swing one leg and then the other out behind you as you jog with your music. Cross pattern your arms and legs: when your left leg is back, swing your right arm in front. When your right leg is back, swing your left arm in front.

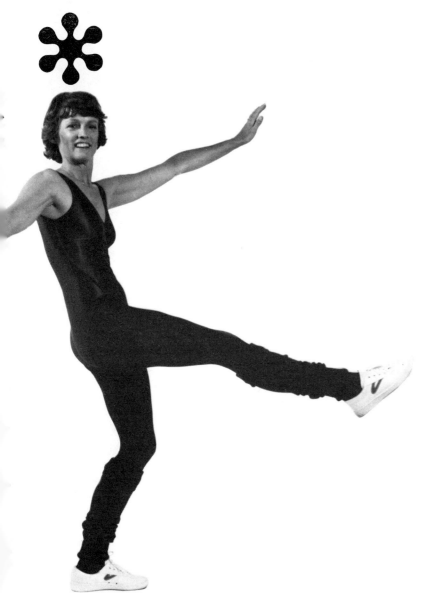

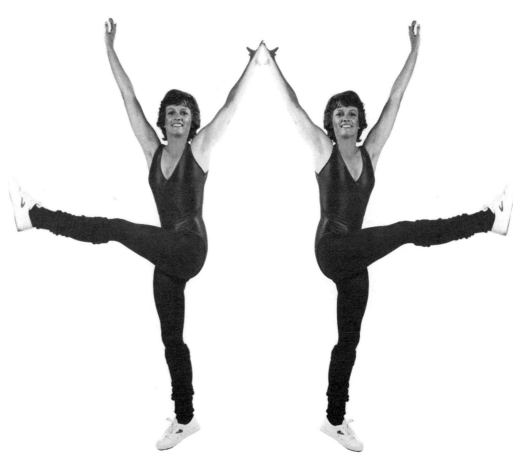

2 Lift one leg, then the other, in front of you as you jog. Continue to cross pattern your arms and legs.

1 *Cross Kick* Lift with your thigh muscle.

2 Keep your standing heel down.

Aerobic High III
JUBILATION

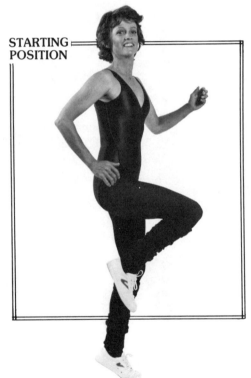

STARTING
POSITION

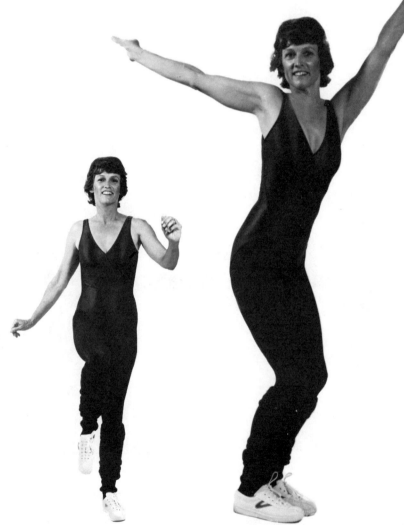

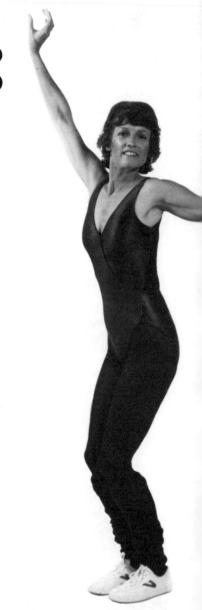

Jog in place. You are in
the home stretch . . .

**Jog Forward
and Backward**
Remember, knees up.

1 **Twist Jump**
Twist your body as
you jump to
the left.

2 Twist and jump to the right. For
a more detailed explanation of this
pattern, see page 49.

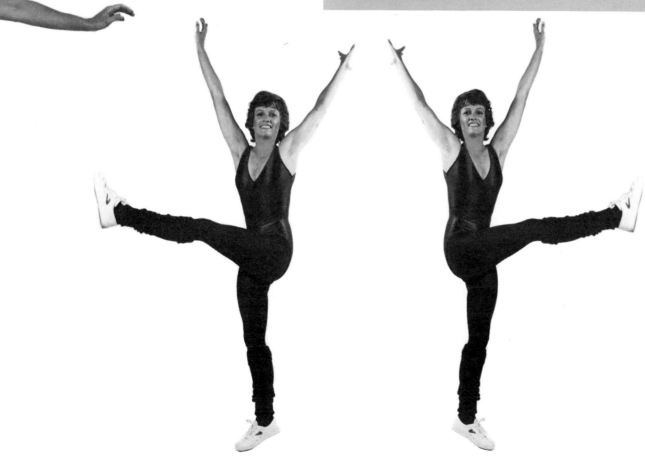

1 *Cross Kick*
Lift your legs . . .

2 . . . and kick across your body.

YOU HAVE DONE IT!
YOU ARE REALLY AEROBIC!
Have a big drink of water and move right into Slimnastics.

FANTASTIC SLIMNASTICS

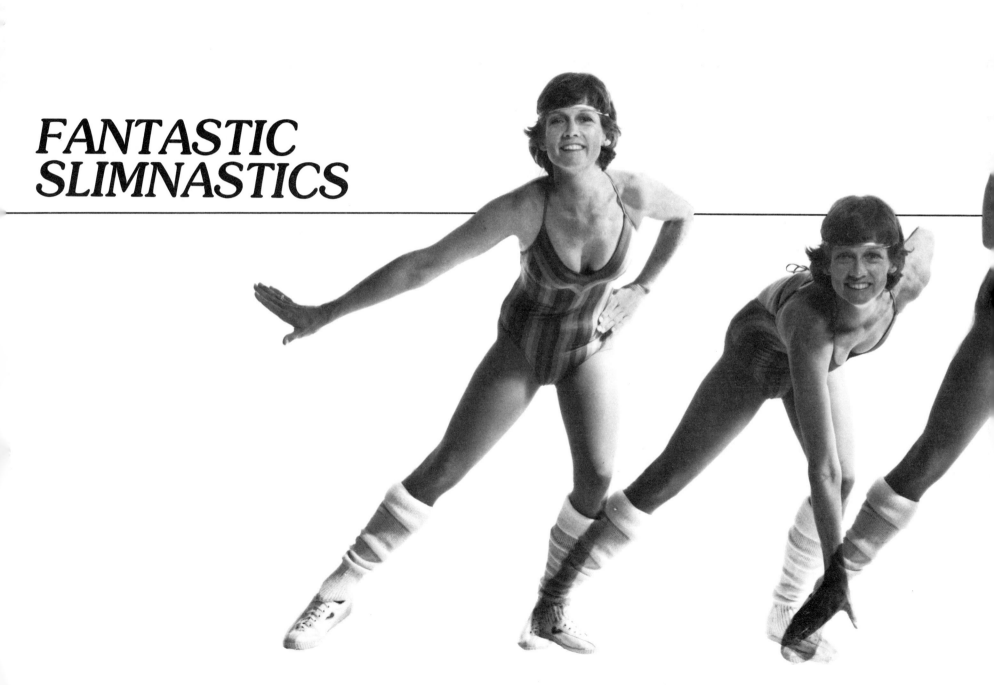

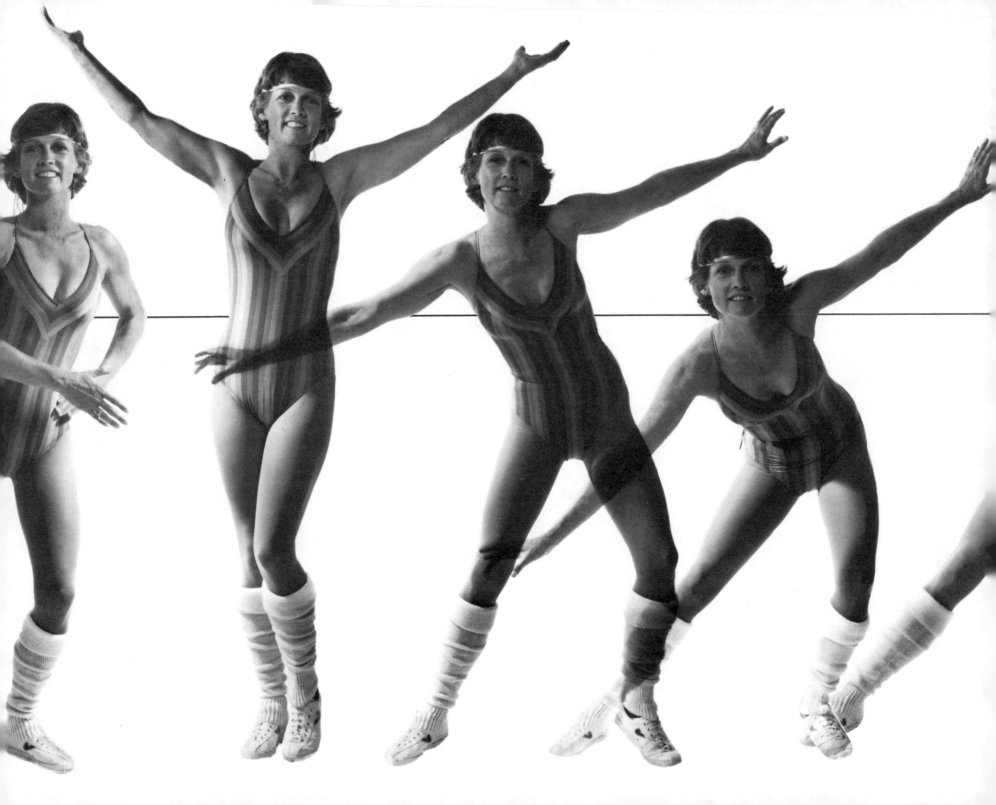

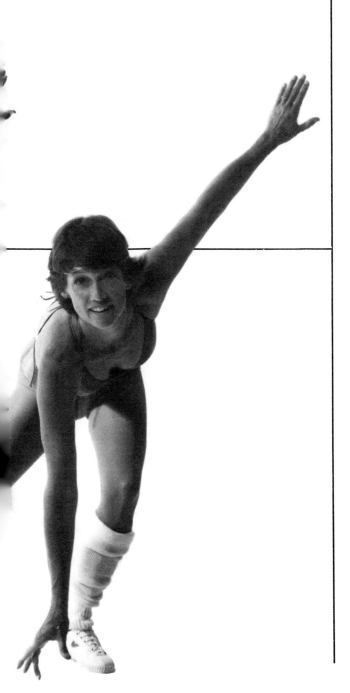

CONTENTS

Start the slimnastics immediately while you are warm and limber. The slimnastics part of the program will tone and firm specific muscle groups as you exercise from head to toe. Remember, it is essential to exercise the total body to burn calories and shed unwanted pounds.

You will feel good during this part of the workout because the earlier aerobic routines have flushed your body with oxygen. Perspiring freely now, you are limber, warm, strong, and really ready to work your muscles. Think of your music as a competent coach, sweating, smiling, encouraging and working with you.

Starting at the Top

*Strengthen your upper body. Tone the muscles of
your neck, shoulders, upper arms, and rib cage.
When you know the exercises and your routine, move
your feet in an easy jog or pony in
place to the beat of the music.*

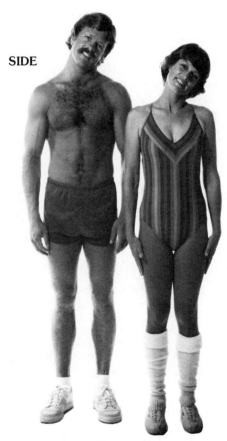

SIDE

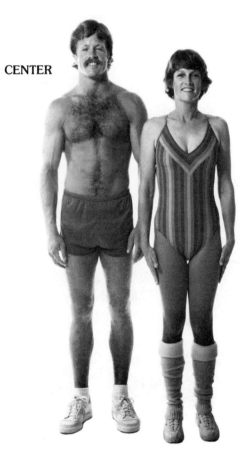

CENTER

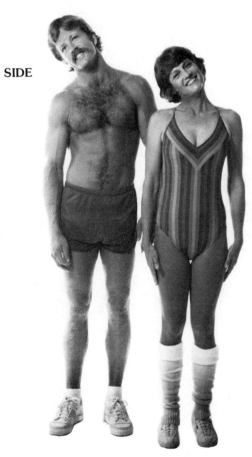

SIDE

1 ***Necking*** Face front with your feet comfortably
apart, your hips and shoulders straight. Unlock your
knees, tighten your buttocks and abdominal muscles.
Keeping your shoulders down, bring your
right ear to your right shoulder.

2 Stop in the center . . .

3 . . . and bring your left ear to your
left shoulder. Feel your neck
muscles relax as you work
with your music.

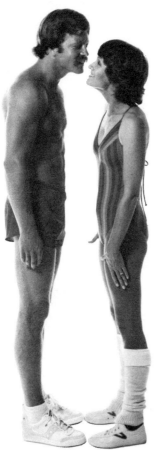

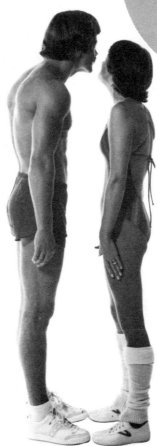

FORWARD

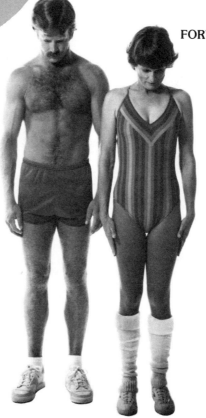

BACK

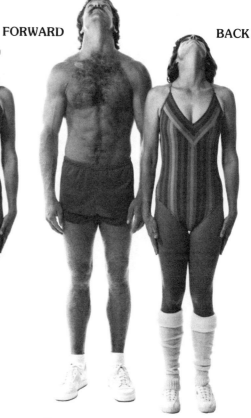

1 *Pecking* Lead with your chin to the right, stretching it out and in for a phrase of music . . .

2 . . . and repeat on the left. This exercise is wonderful for double-chin therapy. Men: Happily, these exercises are built right into your daily shaving routine.

1 *Chinning* Drop your chin to your chest, stop at the center . . .

2 . . . and lift your chin, stretching your neck back.

FORWARD

CENTER

BACK

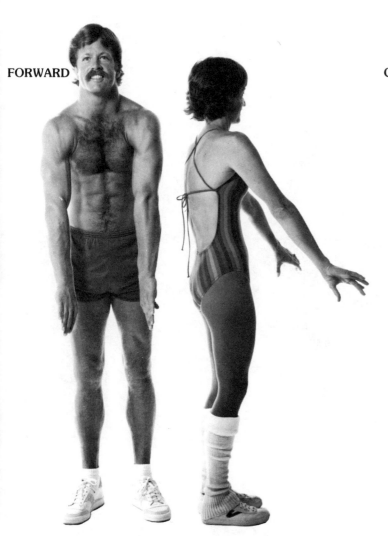

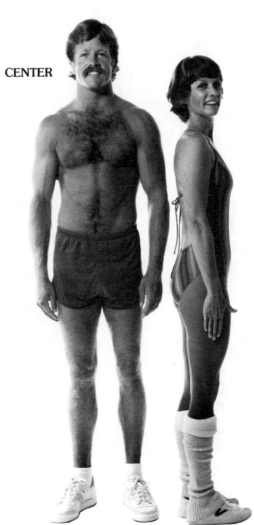

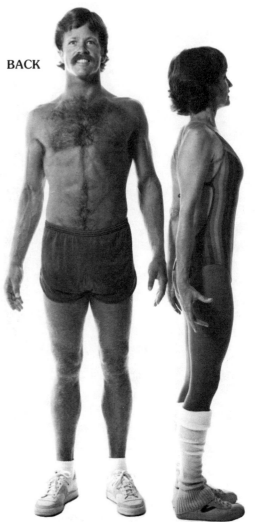

1 ***Shoulder Roll*** Really roll your shoulders forward with your music.

2 Center your shoulders . . .

3 . . . and roll your shoulders back. Roll forward and back to the beat of your music. Feel the tension leave your shoulders and upper back.

How wonderful these exercises feel!

Repeat these shoulder movements through a phrase of your music.

FORWARD

CENTER

BACK

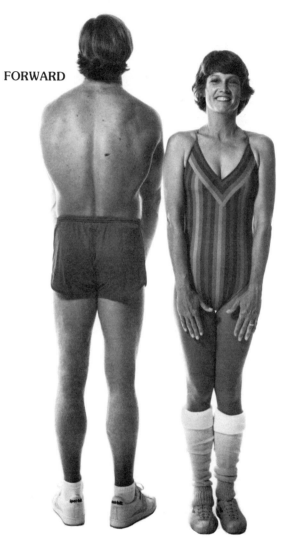

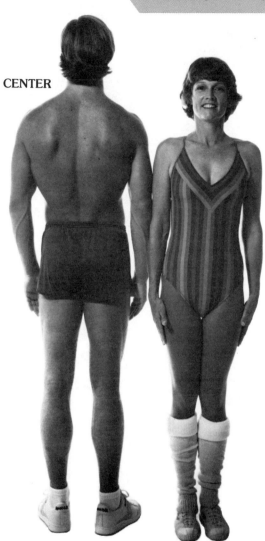

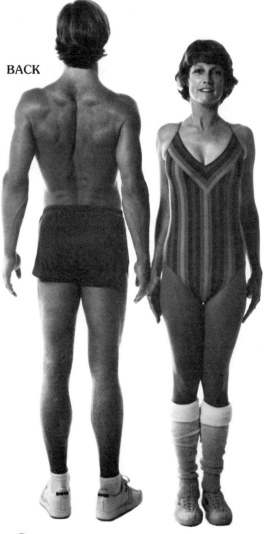

1 *Shoulder Slide* Pull your shoulders forward . . .

2 . . . center your shoulders . . .

3 . . . and pull your shoulders back, keeping your shoulders down and working with your shoulder blades.

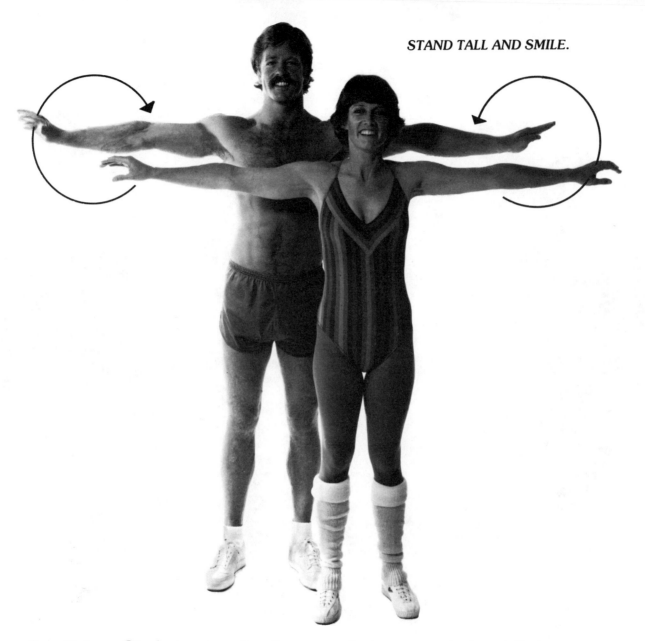

Small Arm Circle Standing tall, pull your abdominal muscles and buttocks in. Make small, tight forward circles with your arms out at shoulder level—palms down. Turn palms up.

Circle your arms backward. Feel your arm muscles working and think about the wonderful toning going on, especially along the undersides of your arms.

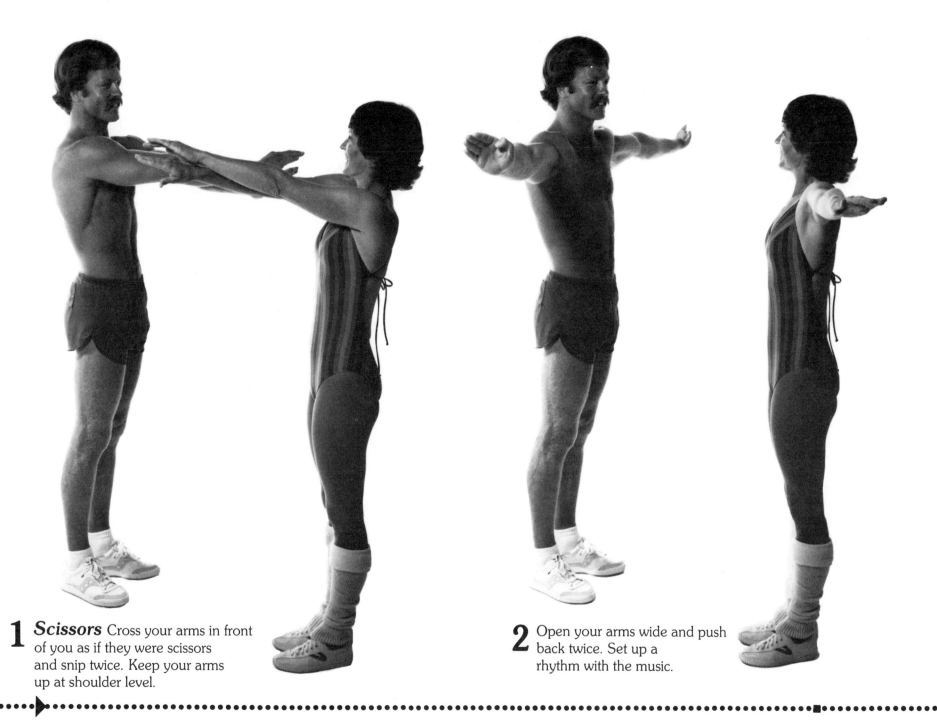

1 *Scissors* Cross your arms in front of you as if they were scissors and snip twice. Keep your arms up at shoulder level.

2 Open your arms wide and push back twice. Set up a rhythm with the music.

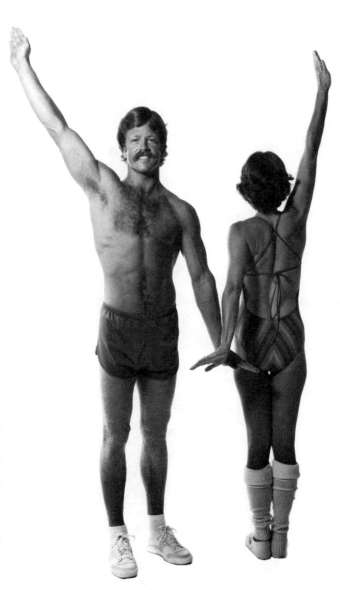

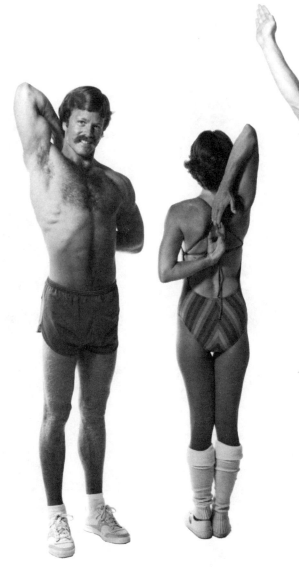

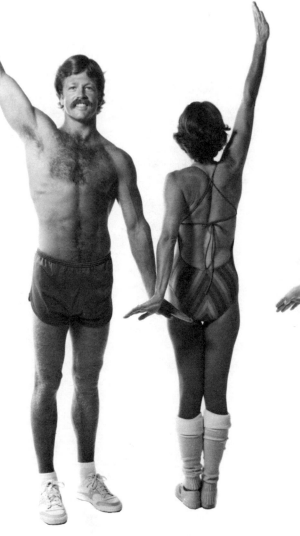

1 ***Diagonal Reach Back*** Starting on your right side, reach up with your right arm and push down with your left. Feel the stretch diagonally from the fingertips of your right raised hand through the fingers of the left hand at your waist.

2 Reach behind you, trying to "hold hands."

3 Stretch back open on the diagonal.

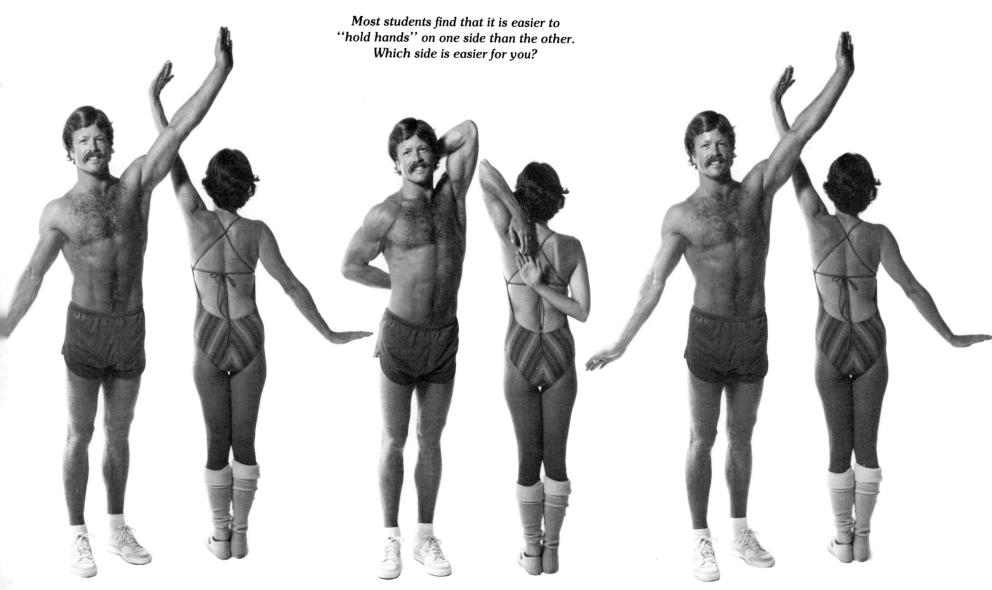

Most students find that it is easier to "hold hands" on one side than the other. Which side is easier for you?

4 Reverse the diagonal stretch.

5 Reach over your shoulder with your left hand and up in the back with your right hand, and try to "hold hands."

6 Stretch back open on the diagonal. Continue to reverse the diagonal stretch and work with your music until you are comfortable with this exercise and enjoy the stretch.

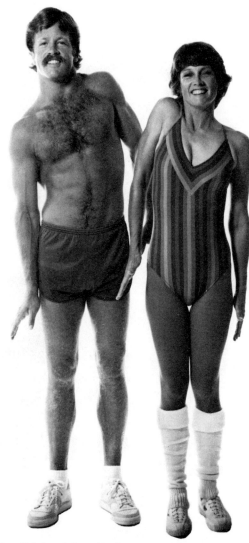

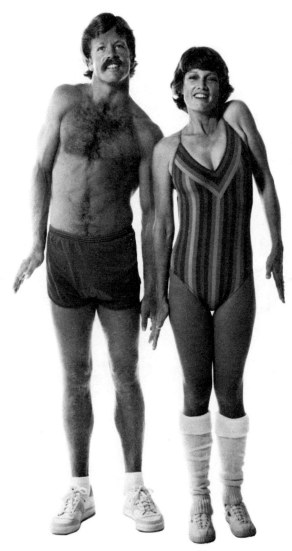

Try any or all of these shoulder exercises at your desk and feel shoulder and neck tension disappear.

1 ***Shoulder Lift*** Lift your left shoulder up toward your ear, relaxing your right shoulder. Lift your right shoulder up toward your ear, relaxing your left shoulder.

2 Alternate shoulders, lifting to the beat of your music.

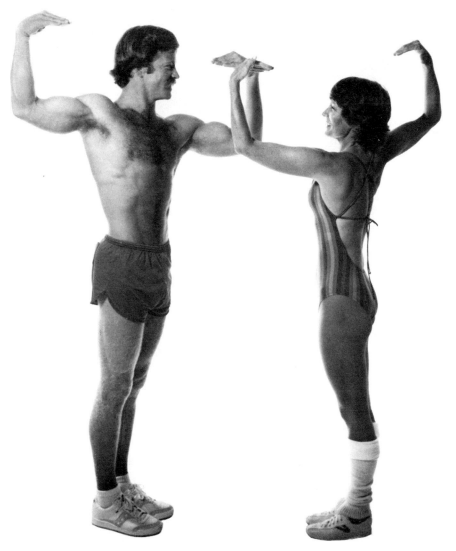
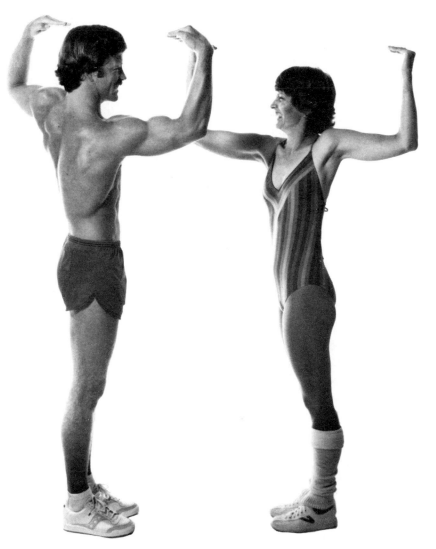

1 ***Egyptian Arms*** Standing in place, pivot your upper body at your waist to the right. Frame your face, keeping your arms up at shoulder level and tightening the muscles of your arms at the farthest point in the pivot.

2 Pivot back to the left. Feel the stretch in your waist and the tightening in your arm muscles. Pivot with your music.

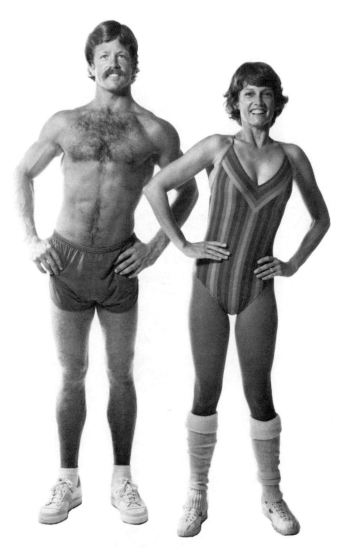

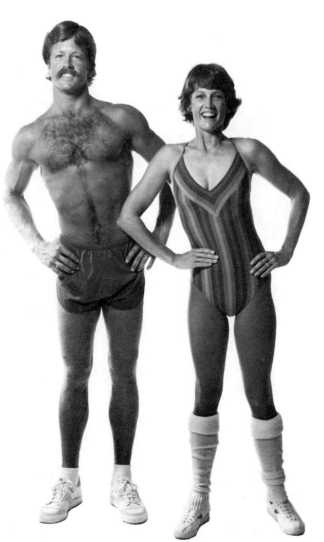

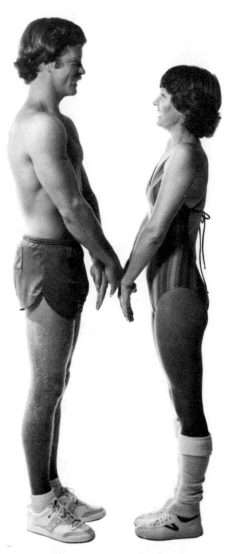

1 *Rib Cage Reach* Pretend you are hinged at the waist. Push your chest diagonally out over your right hip and then relax, centering your rib cage again. Work on the right side through a phrase of music and . . .

2 . . . then repeat on the left side. Keep everything below the waist still. To help you gain control of your rib cage muscles, try this in front of a mirror. This exercise will help you trim away the little bulge above your waist, and you will again see the ripple of your rib cage.

1 *Big Arm Circle* End this routine with a Big Arm Circle.

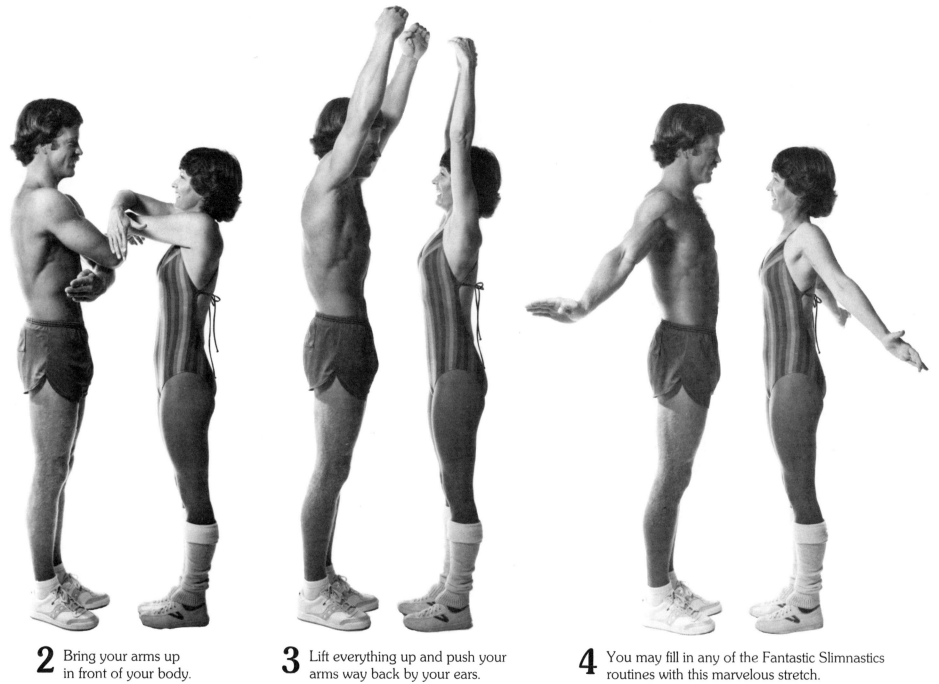

2 Bring your arms up in front of your body.

3 Lift everything up and push your arms way back by your ears.

4 You may fill in any of the Fantastic Slimnastics routines with this marvelous stretch.

Working On Down

Strengthen your upper body and trim your waist. You are warmed up now because you have worked through your aerobic routines, so you can bounce on these slimnastic exercises and benefit from the extra stretch.
Enjoy standing tall "posture perfect."

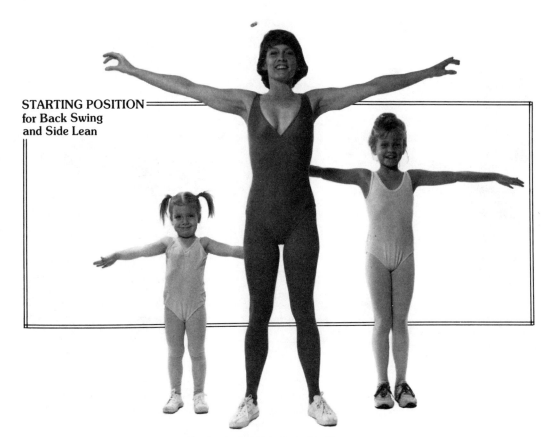

STARTING POSITION
for Back Swing
and Side Lean

WAIST TRIMMER Arms out at shoulder level. Pull your abdominal muscles in. *SMILE. These exercises feel so good.*

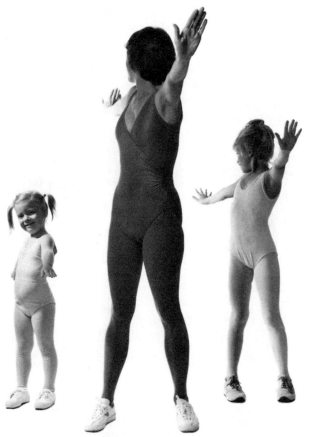

1 *Back Swing* Keep your arms at shoulder level and let your eyes follow your back hand as you swing toward the back. Bounce gently back a little farther.

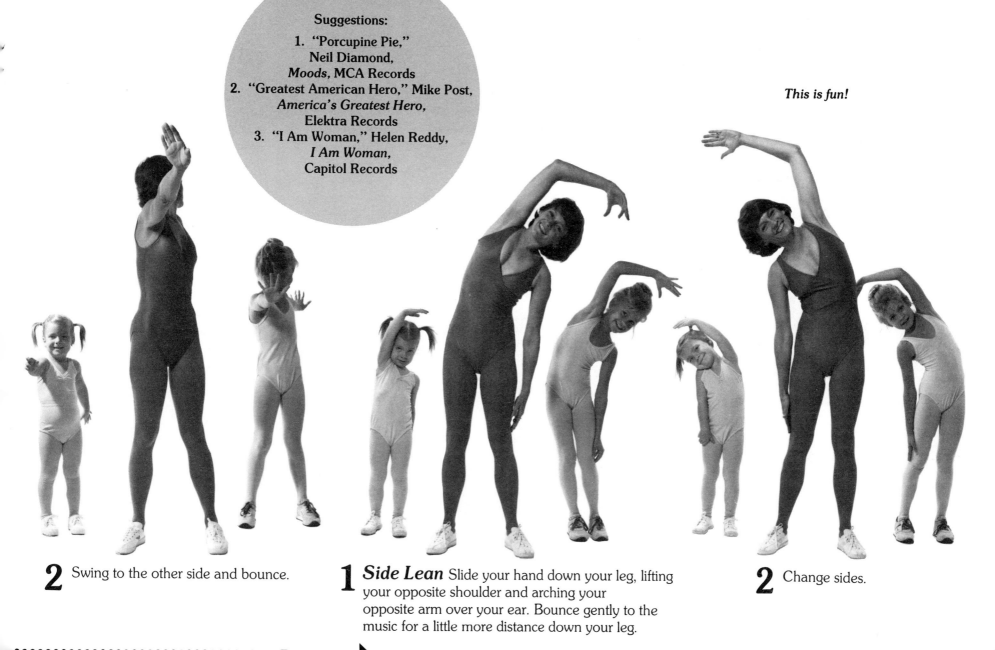

This is fun!

2 Swing to the other side and bounce.

1 **Side Lean** Slide your hand down your leg, lifting your opposite shoulder and arching your opposite arm over your ear. Bounce gently to the music for a little more distance down your leg.

2 Change sides.

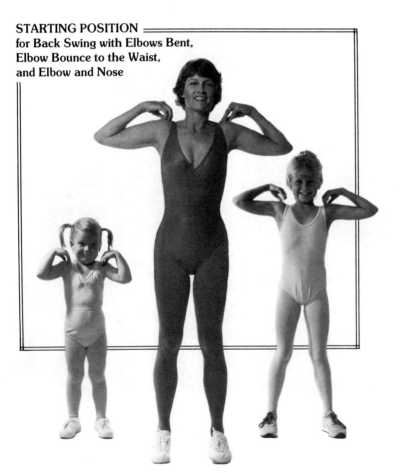

for Back Swing with Elbows Bent,
Elbow Bounce to the Waist,
and Elbow and Nose

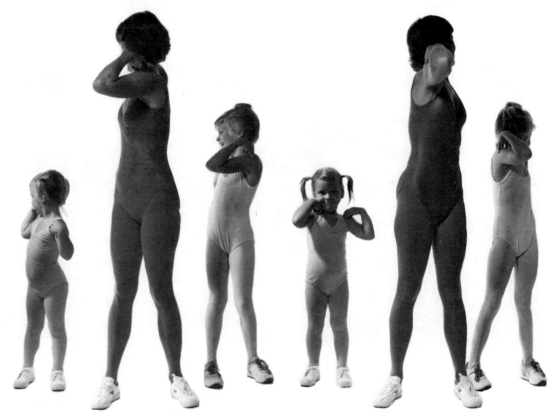

WAIST TRIMMER ELBOWS BENT

Put your hands on your shoulders. Keep your elbows
at shoulder level and stand very tall. Work each
of these exercises through a phrase of music.

1 *Back Swing with Elbows Bent*
Really stretch as you swing
your upper body toward the
back and gently bounce.

2 Reverse direction.

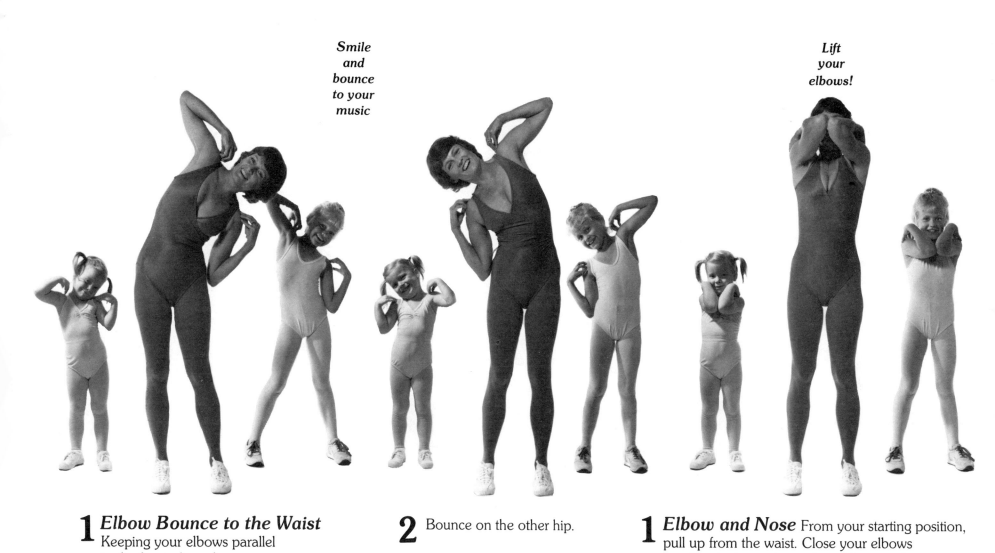

*Smile
and
bounce
to your
music*

*Lift
your
elbows!*

1 ***Elbow Bounce to the Waist***
Keeping your elbows parallel
to the front plane, bounce your
elbow to your hip.

2 Bounce on the other hip.

1 ***Elbow and Nose*** From your starting position,
pull up from the waist. Close your elbows
together in front of your face. No nose showing.
Open and close your elbows over your nose.

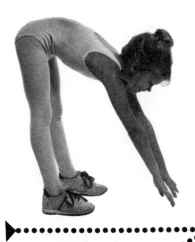

1 *Front-Center-Back Reach*
FRONT
Relax your knees. Lean over at the waist, reaching for the floor about six inches in front of your feet.

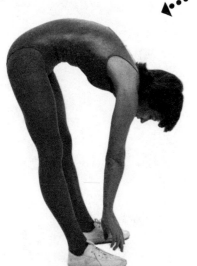

2 CENTER
Reach for the floor between your feet.

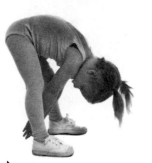

3 BACK
Reach through your legs as far as you can. Try to touch the floor behind you! If you are not stretching to the floor during any of these exercises, never mind. Do your best stretch and one day you will touch the floor.

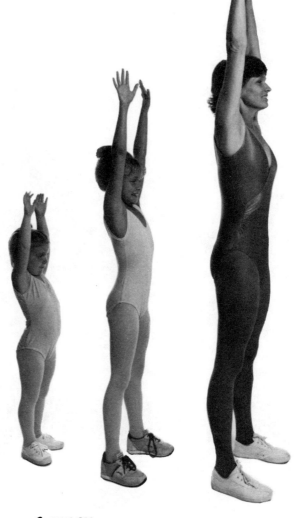

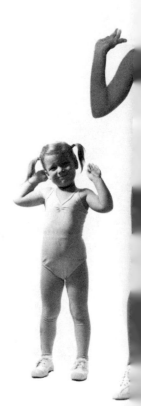

4 REACH
Slowly straighten, lifting your rib cage off your waist. Hold your abdominal muscles and buttocks tight. *The sky is your limit!*

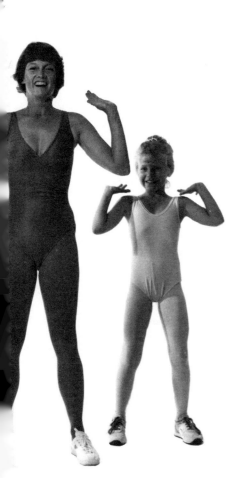

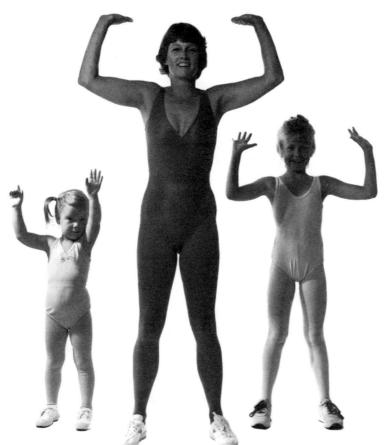

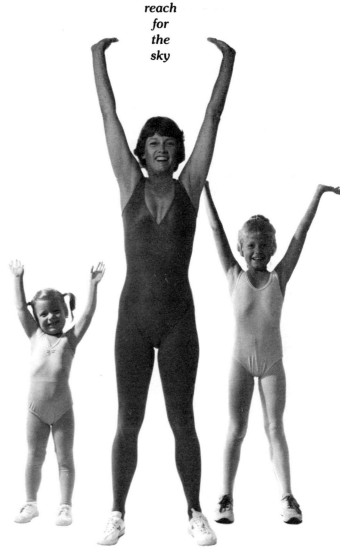

Really reach for the sky

Push the World off Your Shoulders

Face front with your feet comfortably apart. Bring your hands above your shoulders and slowly push up.

2 Resist, but gradually lift. Remember, it can be a heavy world.

3 *You have made it.* As your music comes to an end, repeat this exercise to finish your routine.

Thigh Shapers

Create strong firm thighs and buttocks that will increase your endurance for sports and will work to protect your knees and your lower back.

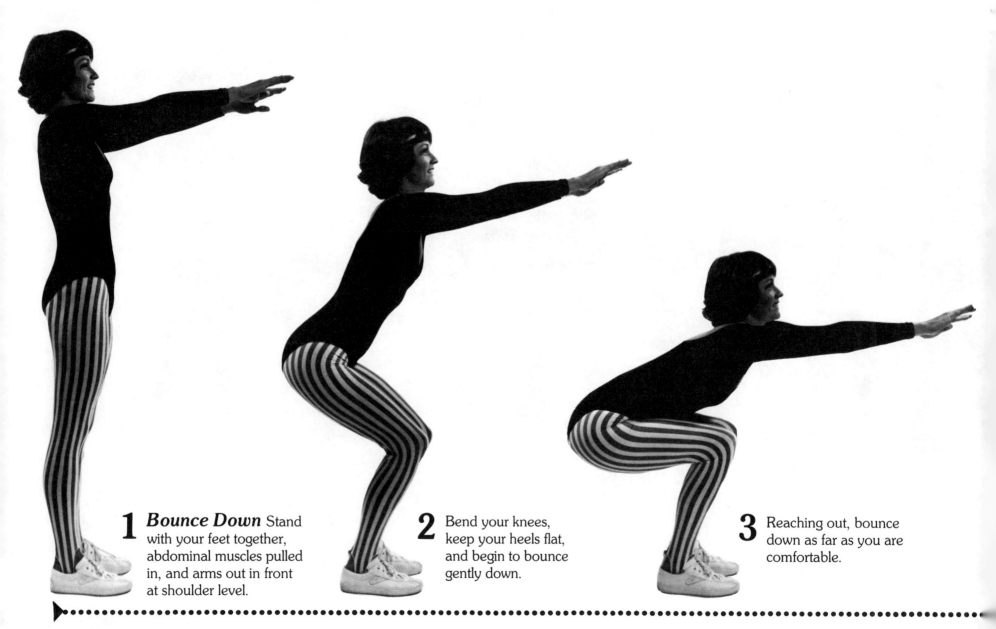

1 ***Bounce Down*** Stand with your feet together, abdominal muscles pulled in, and arms out in front at shoulder level.

2 Bend your knees, keep your heels flat, and begin to bounce gently down.

3 Reaching out, bounce down as far as you are comfortable.

Suggestions:

1. "I'm Gonna Be a Country Girl Again," Buffy St. Marie, *I'm Gonna Be a Country Girl Again*, Vanguard Records
2. "Knock Three Times," Tony Orlando and Dawn, *Greatest Hits*, Arista Records
3. "Make Me a Memory," Grover Washington, Jr., *Winelight*, Warner Brothers Records

1 ***Racing Stretch*** On all fours, extend your right leg back. Keep your left supporting leg straight up and down under your chest and your left foot flat. Gently bounce your groin area toward the floor.

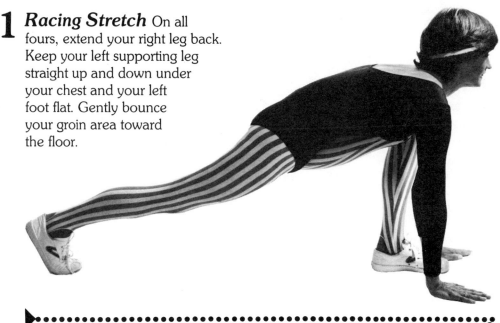

2 Push back, straightening your left knee. Keeping your feet parallel, bounce toward your heel. Change legs slowly or with a jump change. Extend the left leg back and repeat the stretch on the left side.

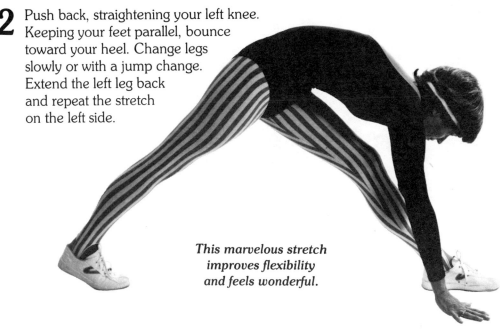

This marvelous stretch improves flexibility and feels wonderful.

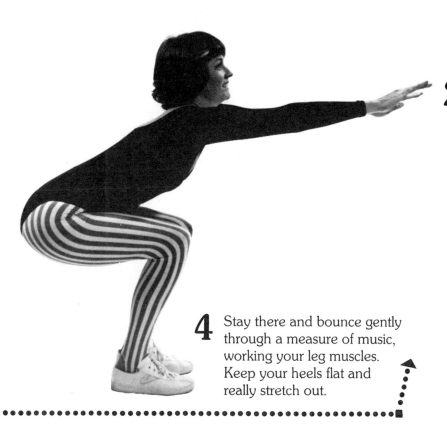

4 Stay there and bounce gently through a measure of music, working your leg muscles. Keep your heels flat and really stretch out.

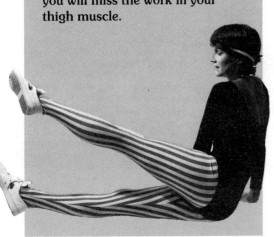

1 ***The Killer Thigh Lift***
Sit down and extend your legs
together out in front.
Keep both cheeks of your
buttocks firmly on the floor.
Place your hands on
the floor by your
left side.

2 Pointing your toes, lift and lower your right
leg to the end of the musical phrase.
Flex your right foot and lift and lower.
Change hands to the right and lift your
left leg, toes pointed, and then lift
with a foot flexed.
Feel the muscles of the
upper thigh working
and toning.

1 ***Big Toe-Little Toe***
Do a Big Arm Circle,
lifting your back so you
are sitting up straight.
Put your hands on either
side of your body.

2 Lift your
right leg.

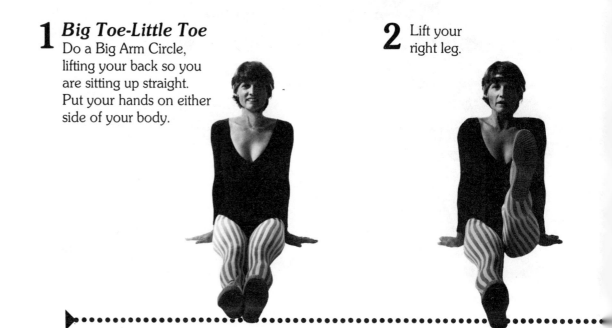

1 *The Killer-Diller Thigh Lift* Do a Big Arm Circle to straighten your back.

2 Sandwich your hands on the small of your back and separate your feet by about twelve inches.

3 Lift and lower your left leg through a measure of music and then lift and lower your right leg. Point your toes and lift, and then flex your foot and lift. Really work your thighs until your muscles feel warm. Try to keep lifting until the end of your musical phrase.

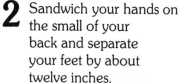

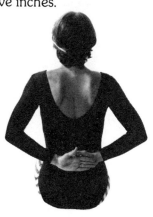

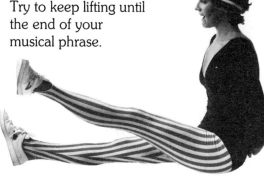

ADVANCED

Move on to **Big Toe-Little Toe.**

3 Swing it over your left and . . .

4 . . . touch your big toe to the floor.

5 Lift your leg back and open, touching your little toe to the floor. The work for your thighs is in the lift, so really stretch out your leg and go for the height. Exercise through a musical phrase with your right leg, and then change to your left leg.

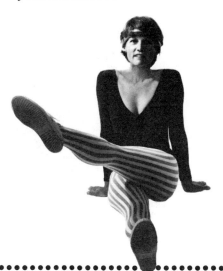

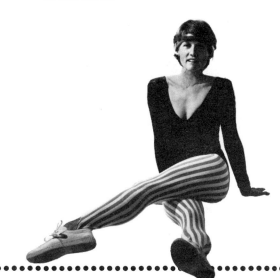

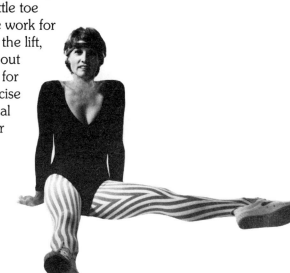

1 ***V Stretch*** Sit with your knees bent, feet on the floor. Reach your arms up, straightening your back.

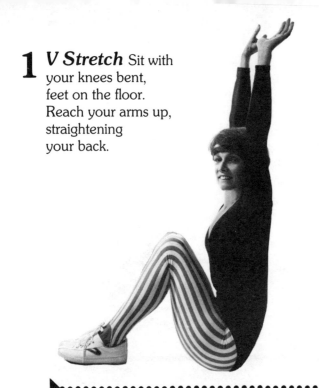

2 Put your hands to the floor on either side of your body. Softly touch your toes to the floor . . .

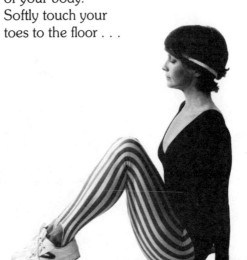

3 . . . and then extend your legs, straightening your knees.

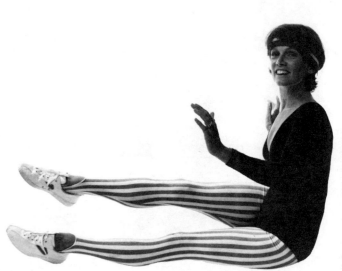

1 ***Hip Walk*** Lift your hips as you "walk" forward and backward.

4 Alternate by bending and extending your right leg and then your left.

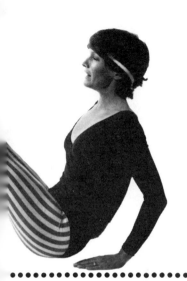

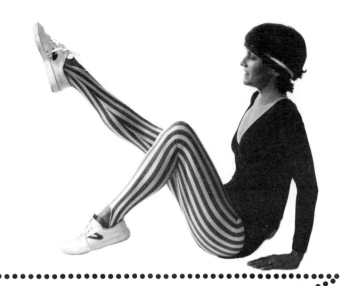

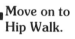
Move on to Hip Walk.

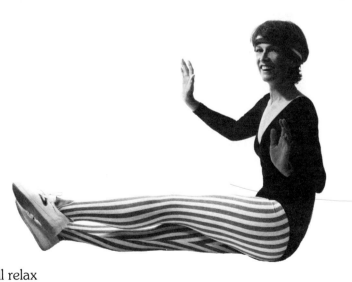

2 Do not drag your buttocks. Really lift. This is fun to do with your music, and the exercise will relax your thigh muscles.

3 End with a Big Arm Circle, sitting tall.

You look terrific!

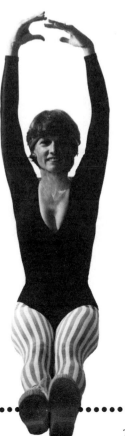

Push-ups and -downs

Firm, strengthen, and tone your upper arms, chest muscles, lower back, buttocks, and thighs. The versatility of these exercises is exciting. For so long a "men-only" exercise, push-ups will build much-needed upper-body strength for women also. Push-ups are marvelous for sculpting your figure. If you are big-busted, push-ups strengthen your supporting chest muscles and prevent sagging. If you are small-busted, push-ups develop the chest muscles, giving your breasts new cleavage and width. The carefully controlled letting down is as important as the push-up, and the push-up itself will develop as your strength increases. Work on your body alignment and control. Work for quality in this exercise, not quantity.

Suggestions:

1. "Hopelessly Devoted to You," Olivia Newton-John, *Grease,* RSO Records
2. "Jack and Diane," John Cougar, *American Fool,* Riva Records
3. "Can't Smile Without You," Barry Manilow, *Greatest Hits,* Arista Records

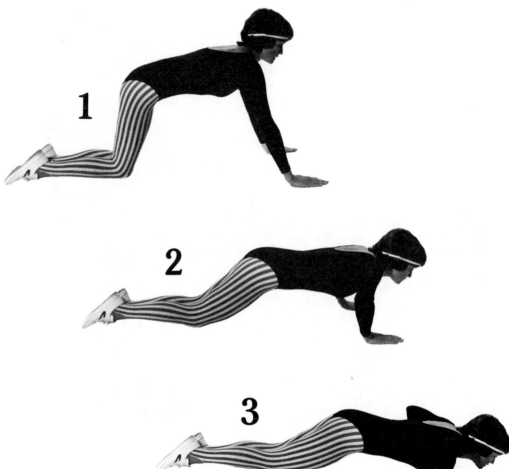

1 ***Push-up*** Kneel on your hands and knees. Place your hands well apart and slightly in front of your shoulders.

2 Keeping your back flat and straight and leading with your chin, lower your body. . .

3 . . . until it is just off the floor.

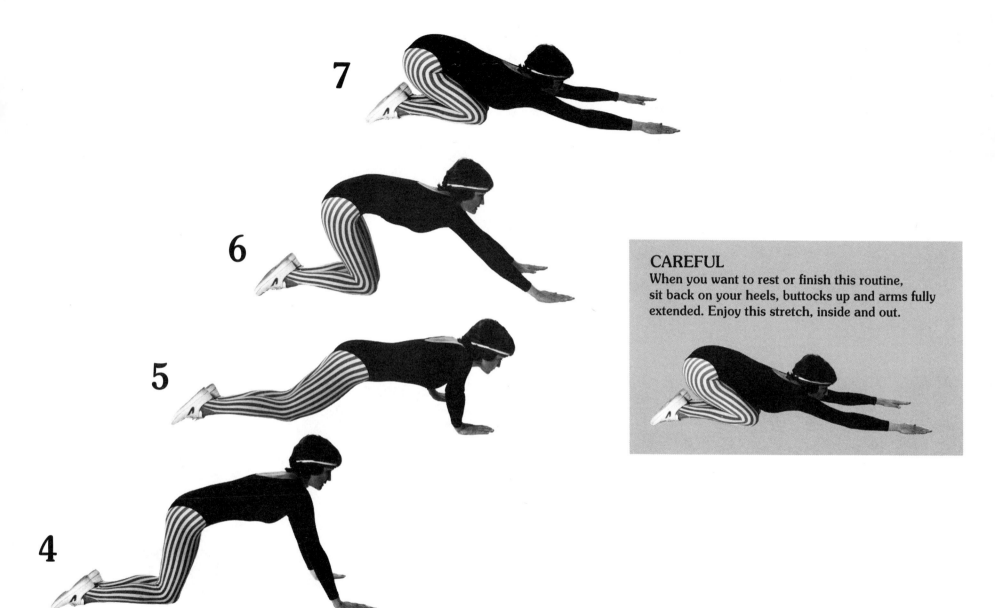

CAREFUL
When you want to rest or finish this routine, sit back on your heels, buttocks up and arms fully extended. Enjoy this stretch, inside and out.

4 If you cannot hold your weight or push back up, relax and let yourself sink to the floor. Get back up on all fours any way you can, straighten out your back . . .

5 . . . and lower again.

6 Push up, pull back . . .

7 . . . and stretch. From this position you're ready to go right on to the next exercise, the Ping-Pong Push.

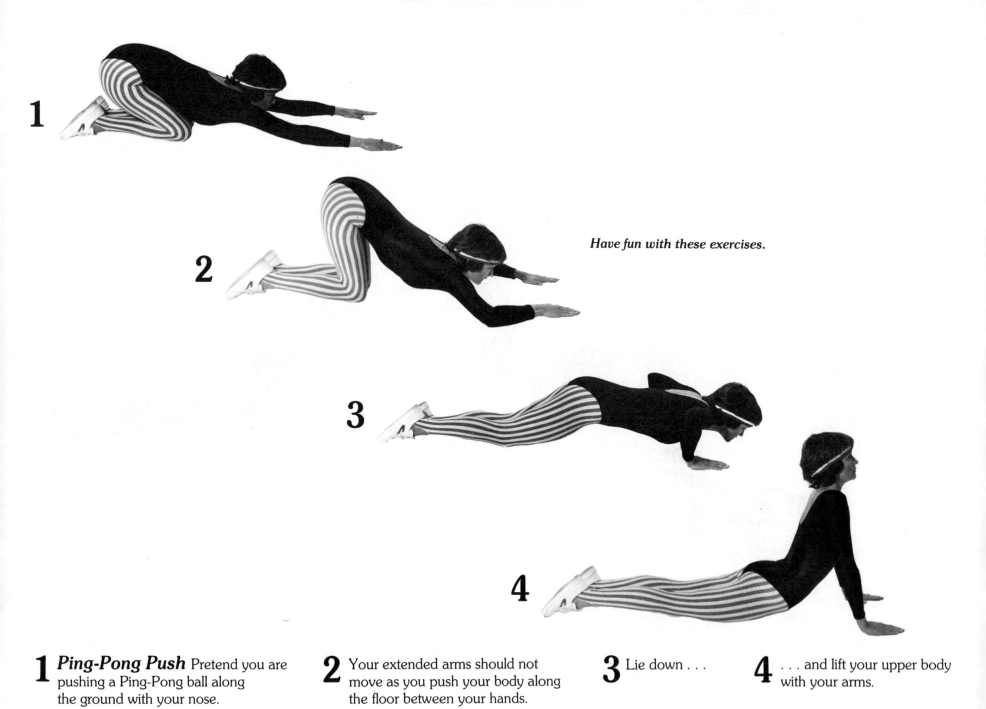

Have fun with these exercises.

1 *Ping-Pong Push* Pretend you are pushing a Ping-Pong ball along the ground with your nose.

2 Your extended arms should not move as you push your body along the floor between your hands.

3 Lie down . . .

4 . . . and lift your upper body with your arms.

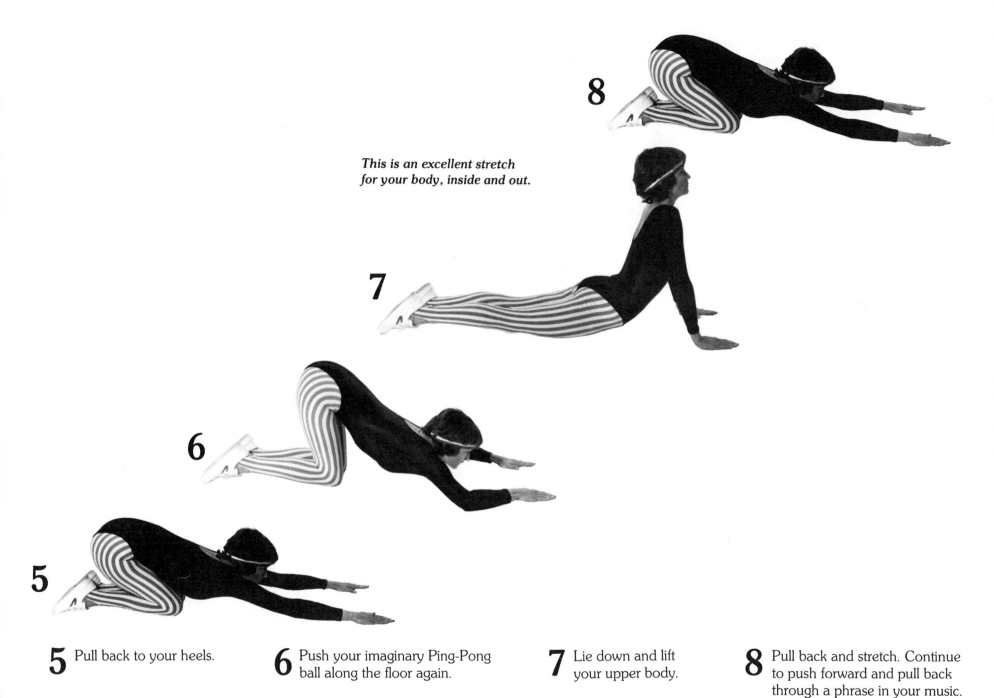

This is an excellent stretch for your body, inside and out.

5 Pull back to your heels.

6 Push your imaginary Ping-Pong ball along the floor again.

7 Lie down and lift your upper body.

8 Pull back and stretch. Continue to push forward and pull back through a phrase in your music.

What are all the wonderful things that
could be stored on your top shelf?
Diamonds, cookies, a fuzzy stuffed animal . . .
You're not tall enough to reach,
and there's nothing to stand on.
<u>*Stretch for it.*</u>

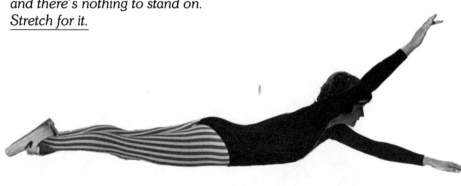

1 ***Top Shelf Reach*** Keeping your
body straight, lift your left arm,
brushing your ear.

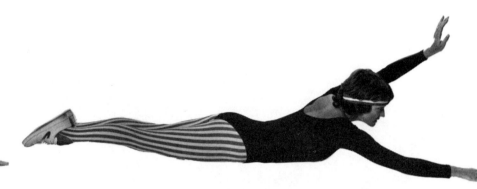

2 Do not roll your chest. Bring your
left arm and then your right arm
up by your ears and reach.

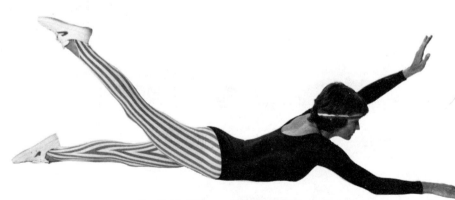

1 ***Lift/Reach Combination***
Combine the Prone Back Leg Lift
with the Top Shelf Reach.

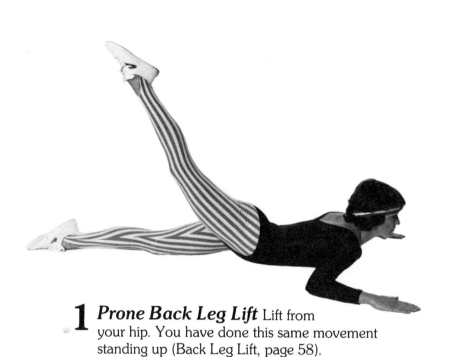

1 ***Prone Back Leg Lift*** Lift from your hip. You have done this same movement standing up (Back Leg Lift, page 58).

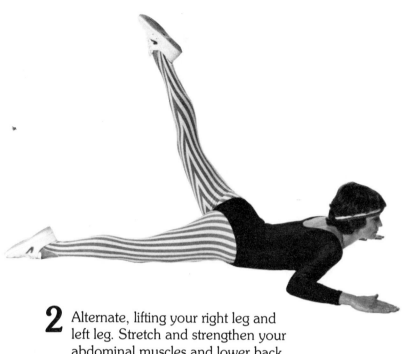

2 Alternate, lifting your right leg and left leg. Stretch and strengthen your abdominal muscles and lower back.

Move on to **Lift/Reach Combination.**

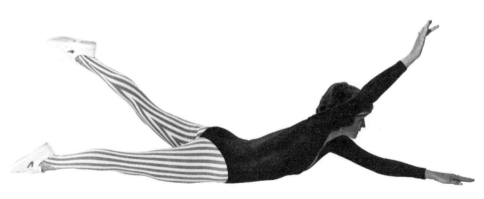

2 Alternate, lifting your right arm, left leg and your left arm, right leg.

This is a wonderful total body stretch and a challenge to your coordination.

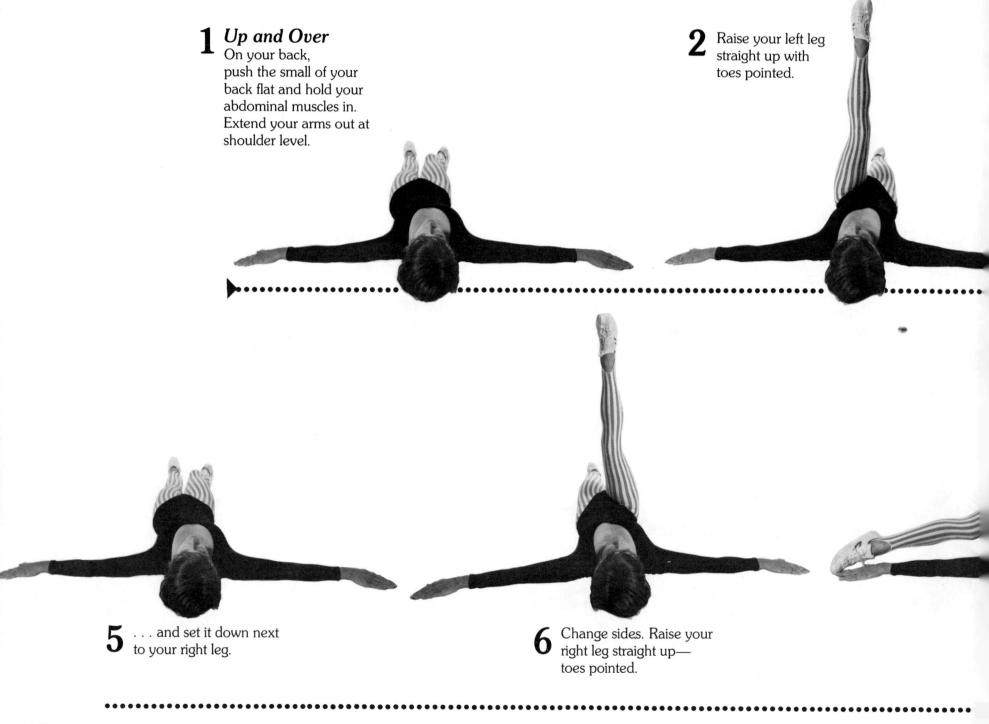

1 Up and Over
On your back,
push the small of your
back flat and hold your
abdominal muscles in.
Extend your arms out at
shoulder level.

2 Raise your left leg
straight up with
toes pointed.

5 . . . and set it down next
to your right leg.

6 Change sides. Raise your
right leg straight up—
toes pointed.

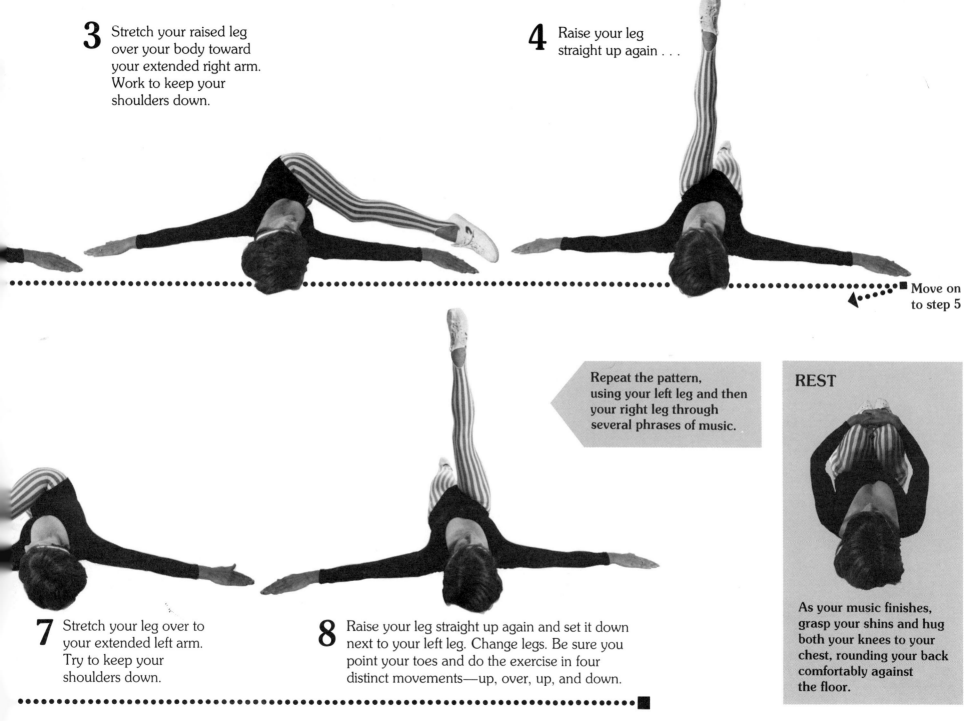

3 Stretch your raised leg over your body toward your extended right arm. Work to keep your shoulders down.

4 Raise your leg straight up again . . .

■ Move on to step 5

Repeat the pattern, using your left leg and then your right leg through several phrases of music.

7 Stretch your leg over to your extended left arm. Try to keep your shoulders down.

8 Raise your leg straight up again and set it down next to your left leg. Change legs. Be sure you point your toes and do the exercise in four distinct movements—up, over, up, and down.

REST

As your music finishes, grasp your shins and hug both your knees to your chest, rounding your back comfortably against the floor.

Leg Makers

Do you want to strengthen and firm your muscles from your waist to your toes? You can do all that while lying down.

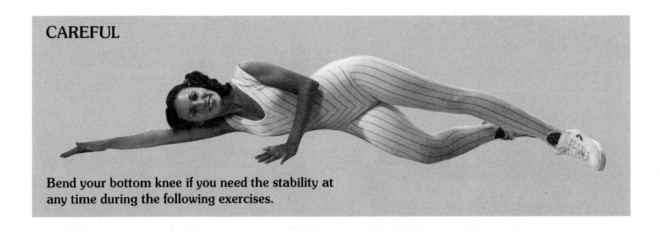

CAREFUL

Bend your bottom knee if you need the stability at any time during the following exercises.

1 *Horizontal Side Leg Lift*
Lie down on your side.
Straighten your body from head to toe.
Pull in your abdominal muscles and
tuck your buttocks under.

2 Lift and lower your top leg,
pointing your toes.
Work through a
measure of music.

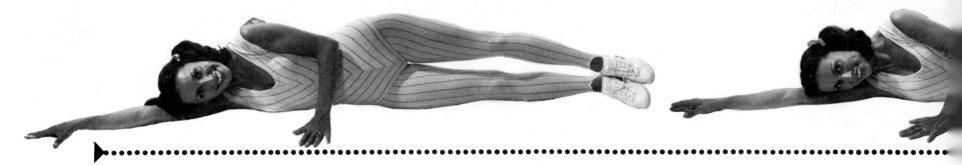

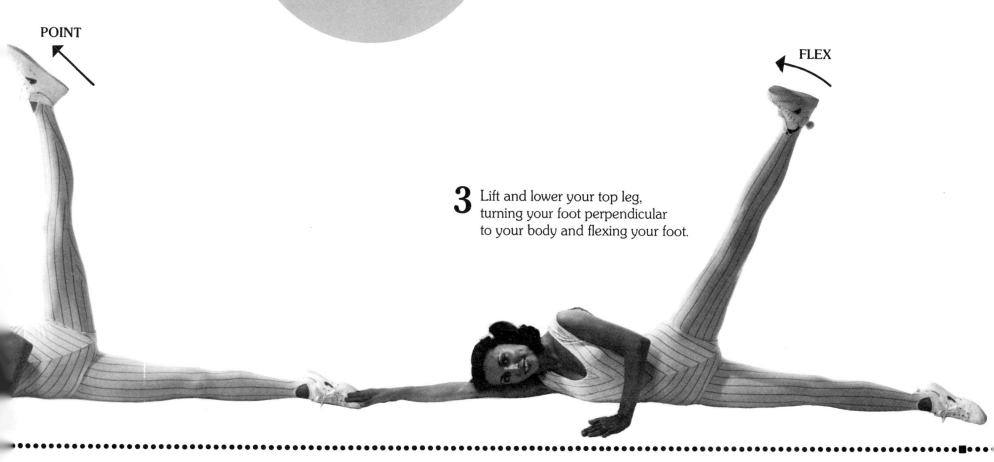

POINT

FLEX

3 Lift and lower your top leg, turning your foot perpendicular to your body and flexing your foot.

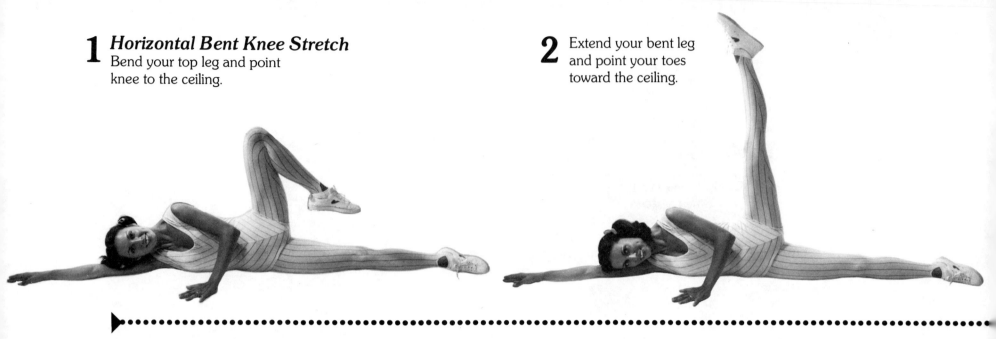

1 *Horizontal Bent Knee Stretch*
Bend your top leg and point knee to the ceiling.

2 Extend your bent leg and point your toes toward the ceiling.

1 *Horizontal Side Leg Lift and Touch*
Stretch out, legs long and both arms over head.

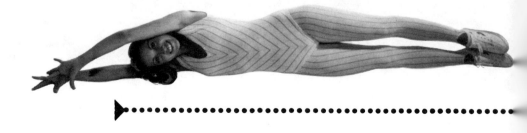

3 Bend and . . .

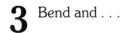

4 . . . straighten your leg as you set it down again. Keep your toes pointed and all your movements controlled. Feel your leg muscles working.

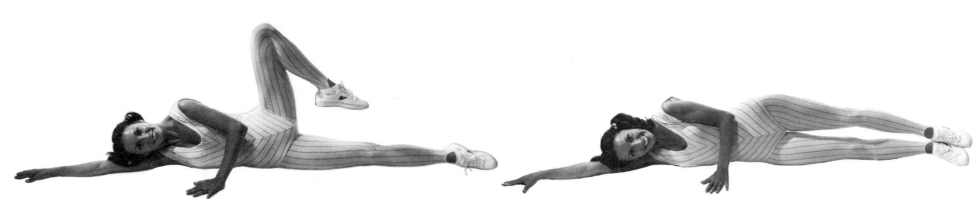

■ **Move on to Horizontal Side Leg Lift and Touch.**

2 Raise your top leg and arm. Concentrate, as this exercise is a coordination challenge.

Shaky balance? Bend your bottom knee.

3 Touch your leg with your hand. Touch and lower to your music.

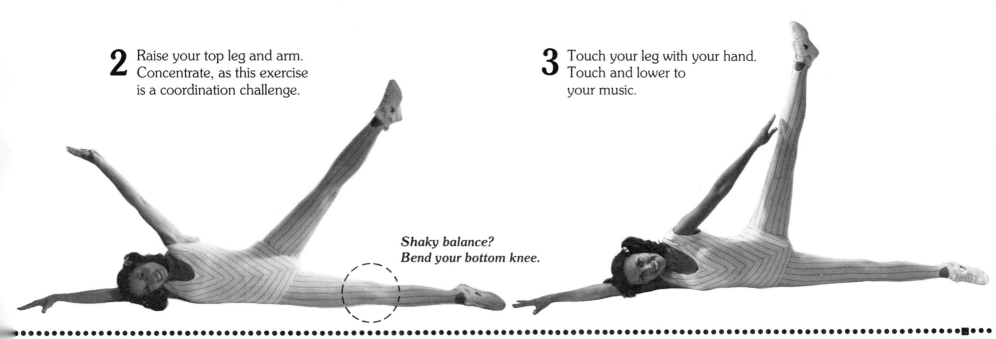

When you begin this exercise, raise your bottom leg two or three times. As you progress, work up to ten to twelve lifts. This is a challenging exercise that does wonders for the hips and thighs.

ADVANCED **1** *Sandwich Lift*
Straighten your body from head to toe. Remember to pull your buttocks under and abdominal muscles in.

2 Lift your top leg up about six inches and hold it steady.

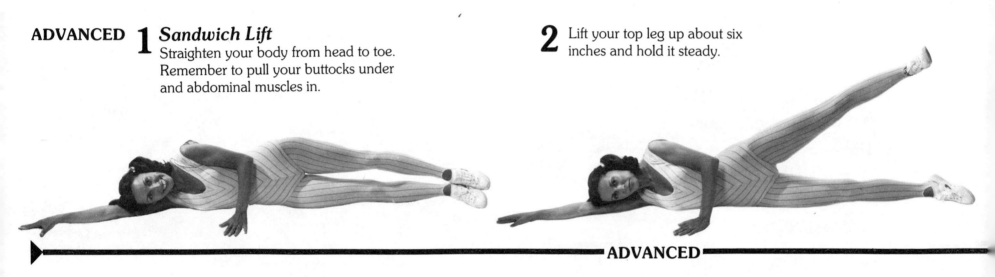

━━━━━━━━━━━━━━━━━━━━━━━━━━━**ADVANCED**━

ADVANCED **1** *Sandwich Swing*
Bend your bottom knee for balance.

2 Swing your top leg forward . . .

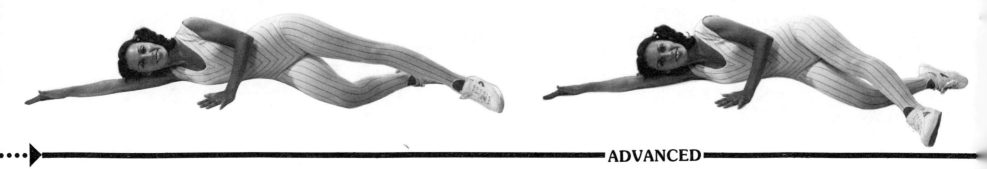

━━━━━━━━━━━━━━━━━━━━━━━━━━━**ADVANCED**━

With your song still playing, repeat the Leg Makers routine, lying on your other side and working your left leg.

3 Bring your bottom leg up to your lifted top leg and down to the floor again to the beat of your music. Think about bringing your thighs together.

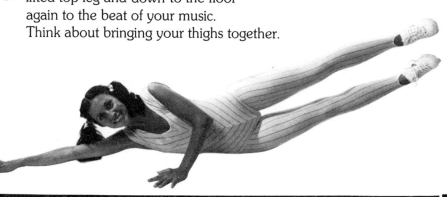

Move on to **Sandwich Swing Advanced**

CAREFUL
If you experience any back strain with the Supine Leg Lift, bend your resting knee before you lift your leg.

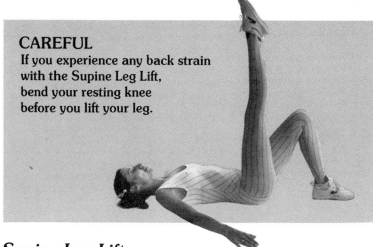

1 *Supine Leg Lift*
Pull the small of your back to the floor.

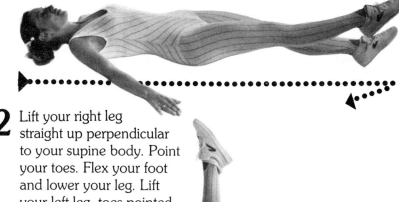

3 . . . and back. Swing and feel the stretch in your lower back and the work in your buttocks.

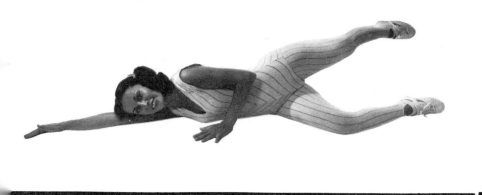

2 Lift your right leg straight up perpendicular to your supine body. Point your toes. Flex your foot and lower your leg. Lift your left leg, toes pointed. Flex and lower. Continue to alternate legs through several phrases of music.

Fancy Fannies

Firm your hips and thighs and strengthen your abdominal muscles!

CAREFUL

1. **Never** let your lower back arch off the floor. Exercising on your back with your legs overhead will work your abdominal muscles. Avoid possible back strain in this supine position.

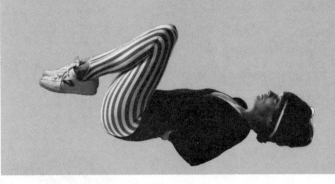

2. **Always** tuck your knees well over your chest. To keep the small of your back flat, slide your hands under the lower part of your buttocks. Lift your buttocks slightly, pull your abdominal muscles in, and hold the small of your back to the floor.

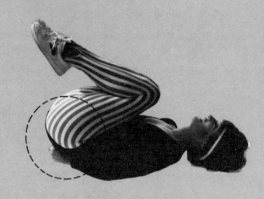

1 *Up and Open*
Place your hands under your buttocks with your back flat and your knees over your chest.

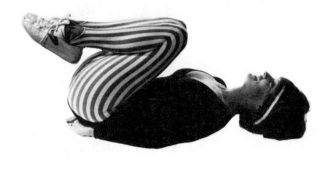

2 Extend your feet above your face, buttocks supported on the backs of your hands.

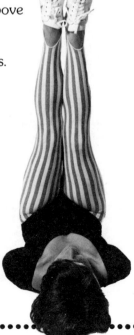

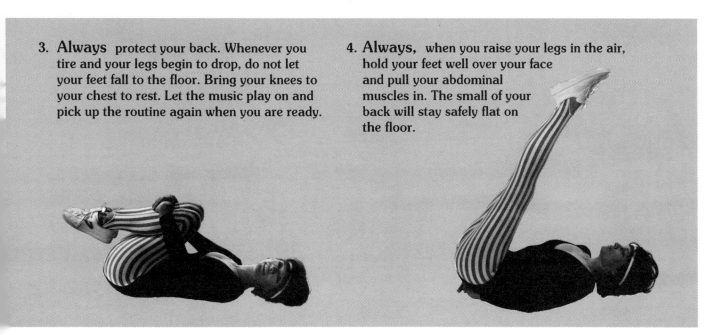

3. **Always** protect your back. Whenever you tire and your legs begin to drop, do not let your feet fall to the floor. Bring your knees to your chest to rest. Let the music play on and pick up the routine again when you are ready.

4. **Always,** when you raise your legs in the air, hold your feet well over your face and pull your abdominal muscles in. The small of your back will stay safely flat on the floor.

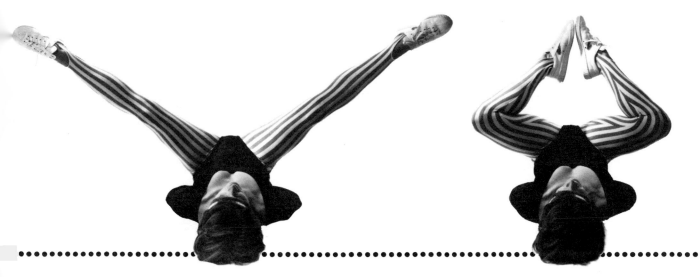
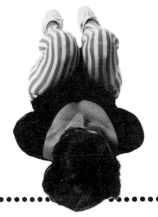

3 Point your toes and really stretch your legs apart.

4 Bend your knees and open them over your chest, with your feet touching.

5 Bring your knees together. Repeat the Up and Open exercise through several musical phrases, enjoying the stretch in your legs and the work in your abdominal muscles.

1 Sole Slaps

Keeping your buttocks supported with your hands, and the small of your back flat, slap the soles of your sneakers, turning your knees out to the sides.

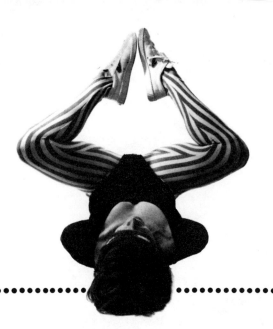

2 Touch your knees

together, turning your lower legs out. Repeat the exercise, working your thigh muscles and rotating your hips.

Move with a bounce.

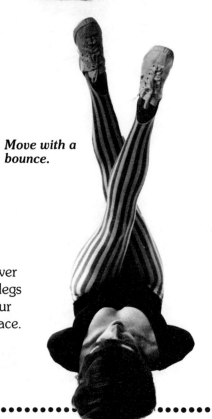

1 Scissors

Slide your hands under your lower buttocks. Raise your legs straight up so that your feet are above your face. Cross your ankles.

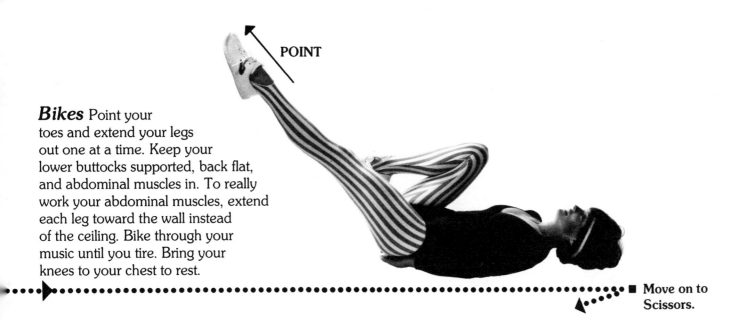

POINT

Bikes Point your toes and extend your legs out one at a time. Keep your lower buttocks supported, back flat, and abdominal muscles in. To really work your abdominal muscles, extend each leg toward the wall instead of the ceiling. Bike through your music until you tire. Bring your knees to your chest to rest.

■ **Move on to Scissors.**

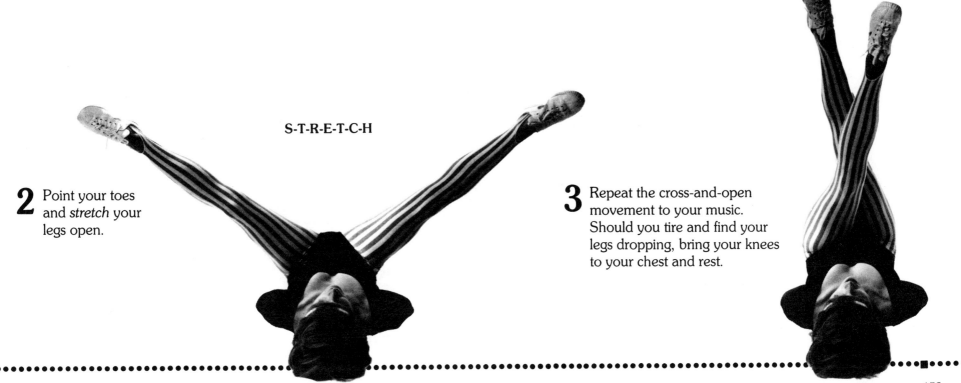

S-T-R-E-T-C-H

2 Point your toes and *stretch* your legs open.

3 Repeat the cross-and-open movement to your music. Should you tire and find your legs dropping, bring your knees to your chest and rest.

1 *Up and Swing*
Lying on your back, flatten
the small of your back to the floor.
Bend your left knee, foot on
the floor. Extend your arms
out to the side.

2 Pointing the toes of your right foot,
lift your right leg up
(imagine that you are touching
the ceiling with your toes) . . .

POINT

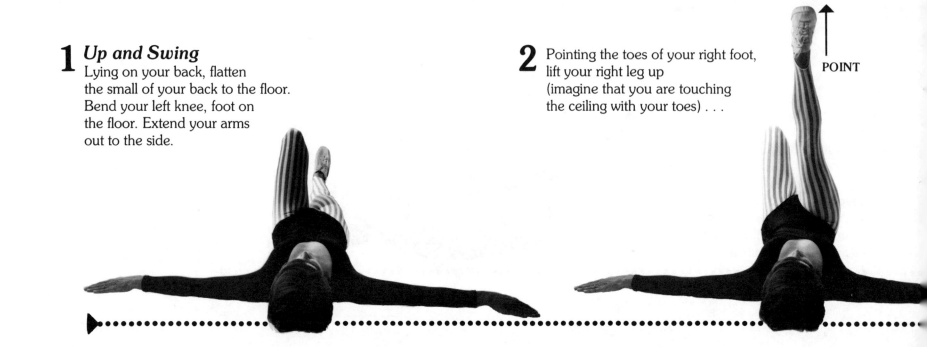

4 Flex your right foot and
swing it out to your
right arm, keeping your
leg about two inches
off the floor.

FLEX

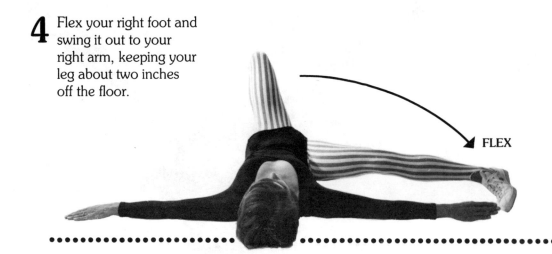

3 . . . and lower it again.

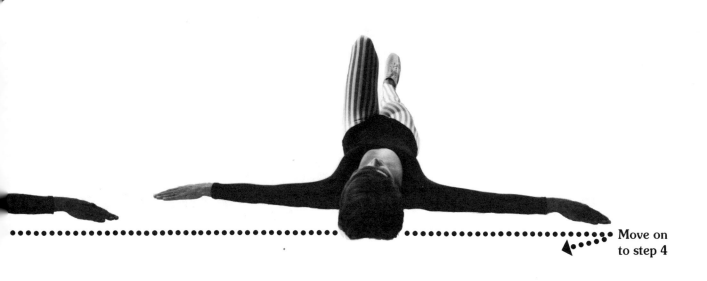

Move on
to step 4

5 Swing your leg back.

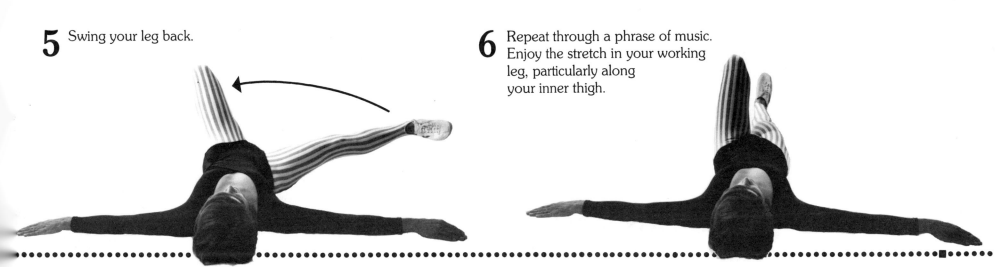

6 Repeat through a phrase of music.
Enjoy the stretch in your working
leg, particularly along
your inner thigh.

As you continue Up and Swing, feel your music with the large movements of this exercise.

7 Change sides. Bend your right knee. Pull your abdominal muscles in and hold the small of your back to the floor.

8 Pointing the toes of your left foot, lift your left leg up and straight overhead.

POINT

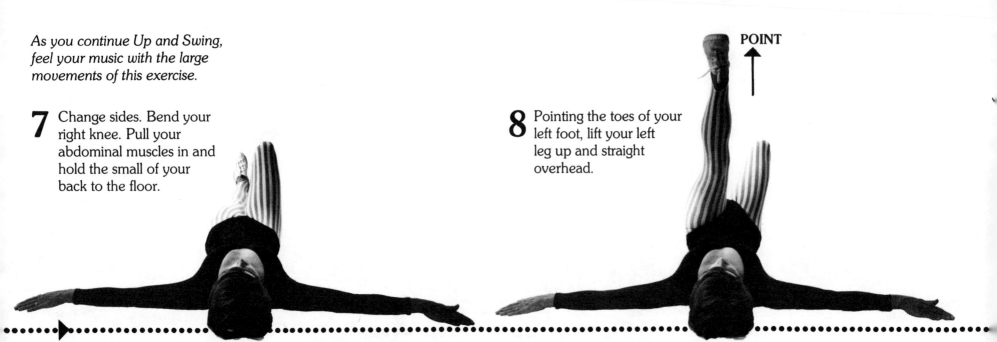

11 Swing your leg back.

12 Repeat through a phrase of music. Enjoy the stretch from your toes to your waist and feel the exercise in your abdominal, buttocks, and thigh muscles.

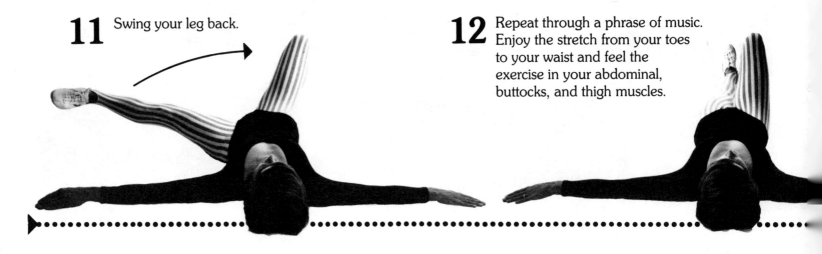

9 Lower your left leg.

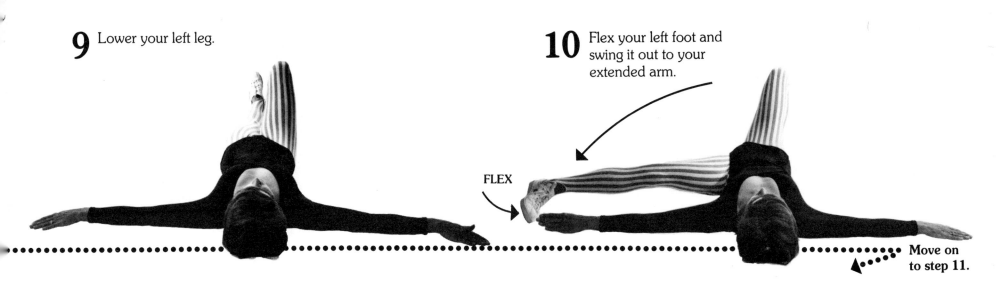

10 Flex your left foot and swing it out to your extended arm.

FLEX

Move on to step 11.

REST
As your music finishes, bring both your knees to your chest, comfortably rounding the small of your back, and rest.

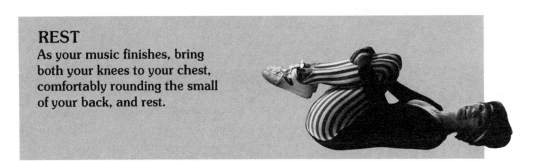

Toned and Tight

Strengthen your lower back and abdominal muscles. Firm your waist, buttocks, hips, and thighs. <u>Really work on these exercises.</u> *They are wonderful toners for an often challenging area—hips, buttocks, and thighs. Exercise with distinct, controlled movements through each phrase of music.*

CAREFUL
If your exercise surface is not carpeted, you may need a mat or towel for your knees.

Angry Cat
Go down on your hands and knees. Round your back like an Angry Cat, pulling in your abdominal muscles and pinching your buttocks together.

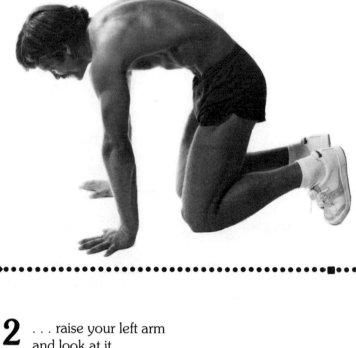

1 *Thread the Needle*
Comfortably on all fours . . .

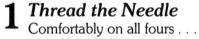

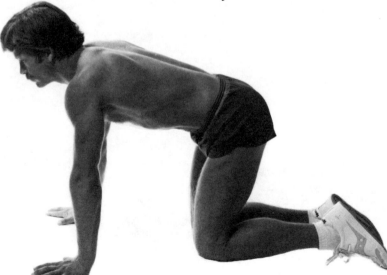

2 . . . raise your left arm and look at it.

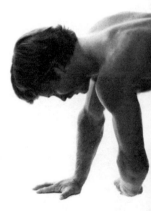

Tired Horse

Let the small of your back sag down like a Tired Horse, lifting your chin and keeping your elbows straight. If you tire at any time during the routine, rest with an Angry Cat and Tired Horse.

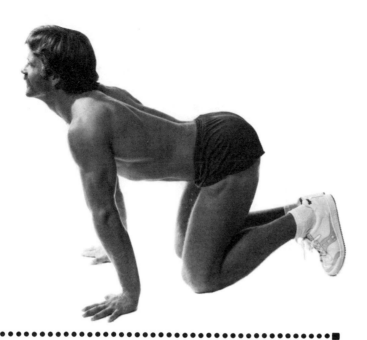

Suggestions:

1. "I Love a Rainy Night," Eddie Rabbit, *Horizon,* Elektra Records
2. "Heartache," Eagles, *Live,* Asylum Records
3. "If You Wouldn't Be My Lady," Charlie Rich, *Behind Closed Doors,* Epic Records

3 Thread it under your supporting arm, letting your left shoulder skim the floor.

4 Follow your hand with your eyes. Return to all-fours position.

5 Repeat through a phrase of music, and then thread the other arm. This exercise is a total upper body workout.

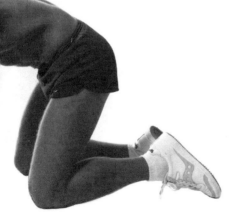

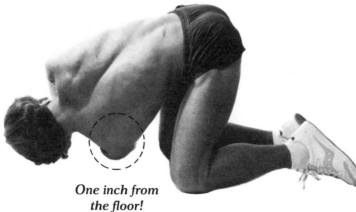

One inch from the floor!

People love Fire Hydrants, because they firm buttocks and hips.

1 ***Fire Hydrants***
Start on all fours.

2 Bring your left knee up and perpendicular to your body. Bending your knee and keeping your leg parallel to the floor, bring your knee as close to your left shoulder as possible.

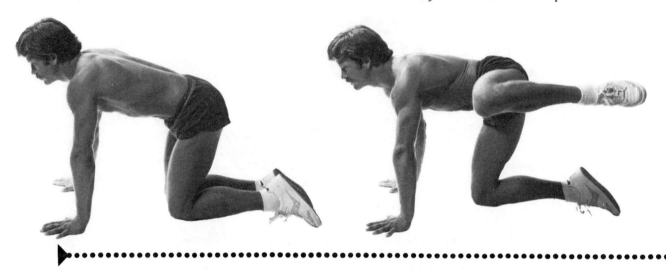

1 ***Swinging Door***
Swing your left leg in front of you. Put your foot down as flat as possible, with your knee straight.

2 Lift your leg.

3 Swing your straightened leg as far to the back as possible and look at it over your right shoulder.
Work on the left leg through a measure of music and then repeat on the right.

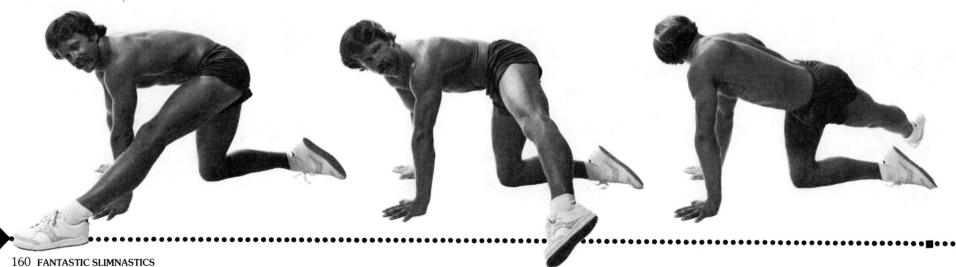

3 Extend your leg out at right angles to your body, pointing your toes. *Extend, do not fling.*

4 Bend your raised leg back in by your shoulder . . .

5 . . . and set your knee down as in the beginning. Continue the exercise to the beat of your music. When the muscles of your left hip and buttocks tire, change to the right.

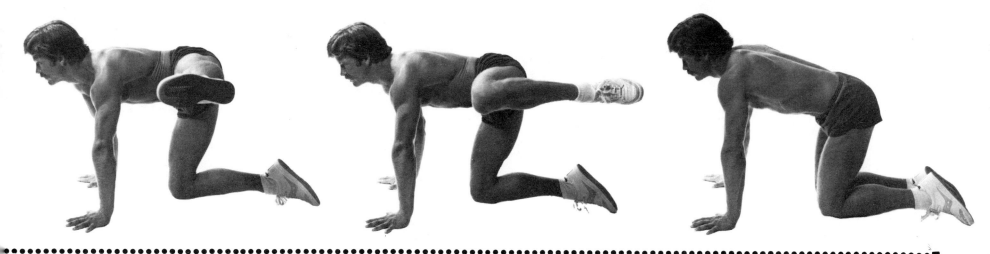

Move on to Swinging Door.

ADVANCED **1** *Swinging Door*
Bring your knee up to your shoulder

Knee to Shoulder

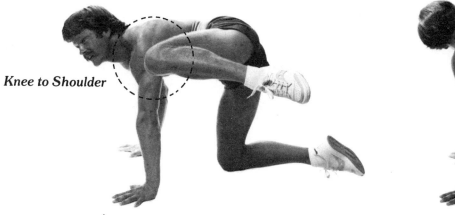

2 and then swing it in the back, looking at it as you swing.

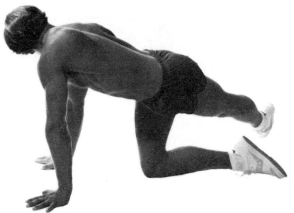

ADVANCED

1 ***Mule Kick*** Bring your bent left knee to your nose. You are strengthening your lower back, abdominal, hip, thigh, and waist muscles.

2 Now extend your leg straight out behind you to shoulder level. Work on length, not height. The stretch is from the tip of your chin to your toes. Work with a phrase of music and repeat on the right.

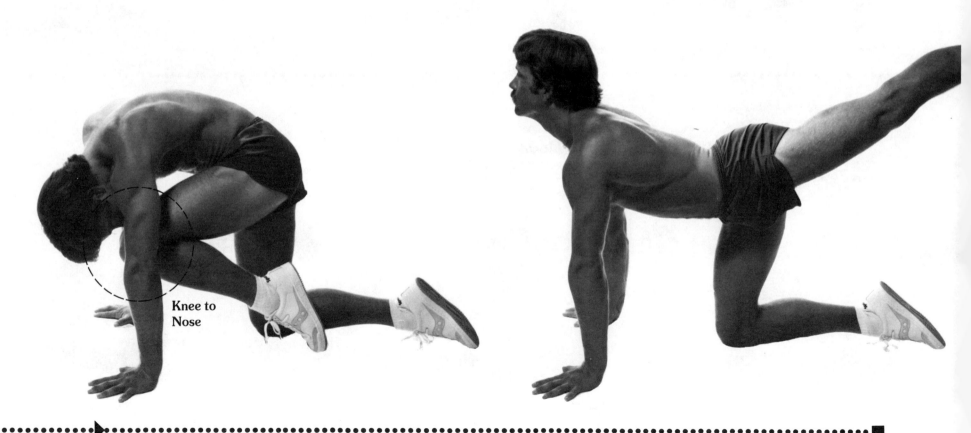

Knee to Nose

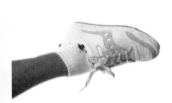

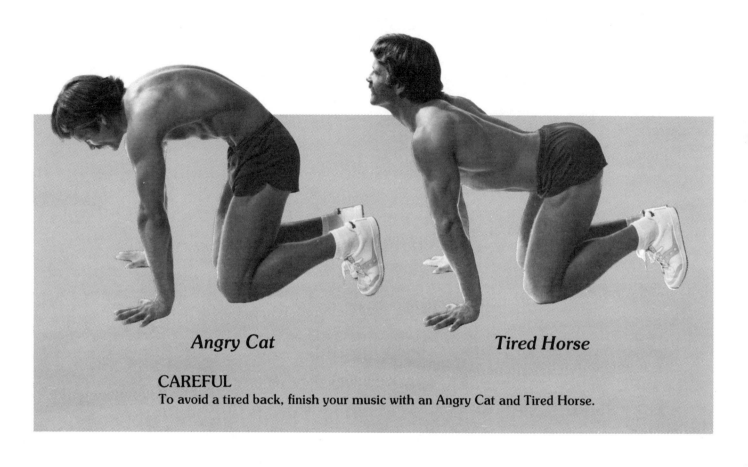

Angry Cat *Tired Horse*

CAREFUL
To avoid a tired back, finish your music with an Angry Cat and Tired Horse.

The Real Sit-up

Tone, strengthen, and firm your abdominal muscles. Strong abdominal muscles will protect against lower back strain, aid with internal processes, and promote the joy that comes with being able to button your pants. Aerobic Slimnastics has three levels of sit-ups. Start with Level I. Work through each level until you find the level that is challenging yet comfortable for you. If you find your feet are coming off the floor as you sit up or that you are throwing your upper body, go back a level until your abdominal muscles strengthen and you can smoothly roll up in complete control of your movements.

The music should remind you of a quiet afternoon.

Suggestions:

1. "Let It Be Me," Willie Nelson, *Always on My Mind*, Columbia Records
2. "Bridge over Troubled Water," Willie Nelson, *Always on My Mind*, Columbia Records
3. "I Didn't Mean to Love You," Helen Reddy, *I Am Woman*, Capitol Records

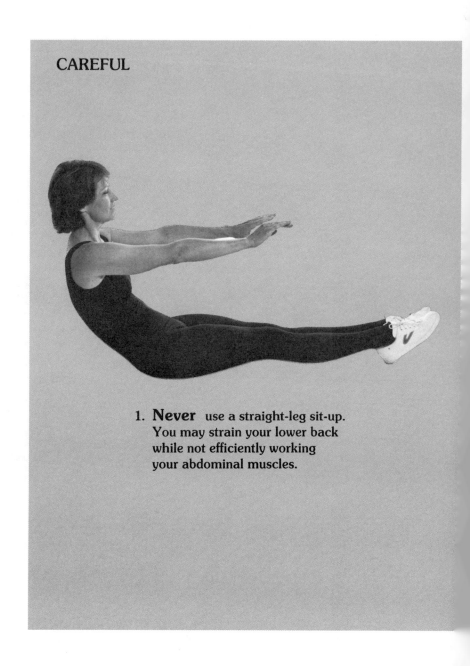

CAREFUL

1. **Never** use a straight-leg sit-up. You may strain your lower back while not efficiently working your abdominal muscles.

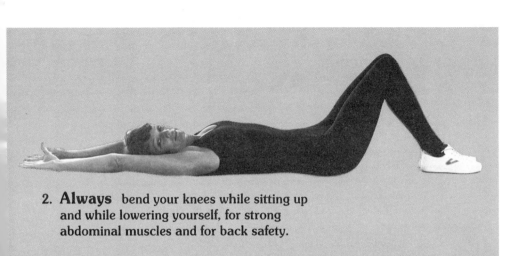

2. **Always** bend your knees while sitting up and while lowering yourself, for strong abdominal muscles and for back safety.

3. **Never** let your feet come off the floor when doing sit-ups. If they do, you are not safely working your abdominal muscles, and the exercise that you are doing is too difficult for you. Having a buddy hold your feet only masks the problem of weak abdominals and creates a possibility of lower back discomfort. Work together with me, and soon your abdominal muscles will be strong enough to do The Real Sit-up without straining your back.

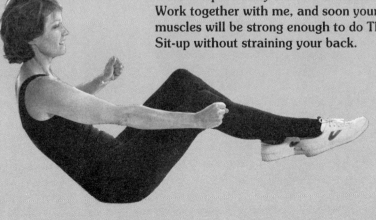

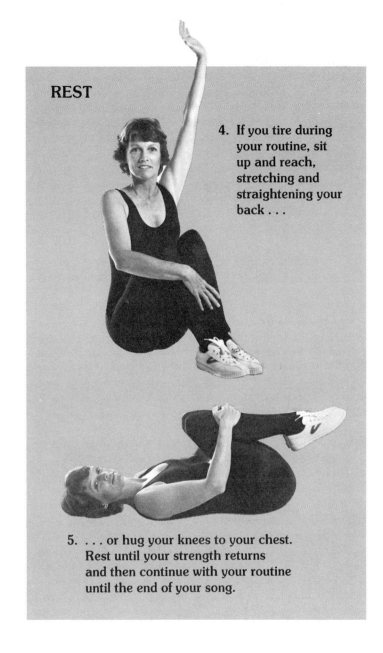

REST

4. If you tire during your routine, sit up and reach, stretching and straightening your back . . .

5. . . . or hug your knees to your chest. Rest until your strength returns and then continue with your routine until the end of your song.

LEVEL I SIT-UP

If you are new to sit-ups or if you have any history of back problems, Level I is for you!

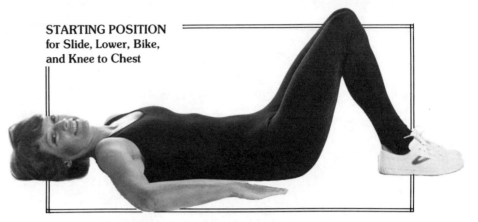

STARTING POSITION for Slide, Lower, Bike, and Knee to Chest

Start flat on your back with your knees bent and your feet flat on the floor.

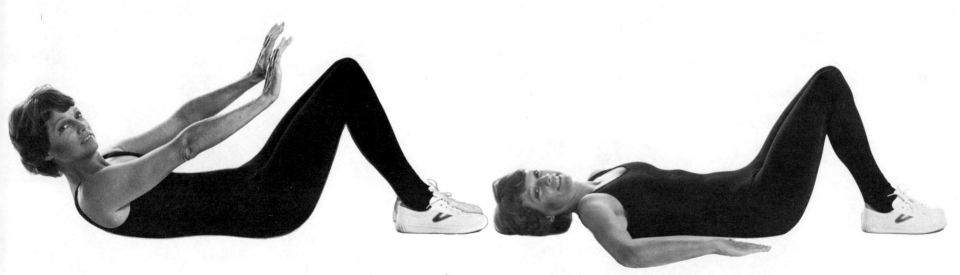

Slide Rolling your chin to your chest and lifting your shoulders, slide your hands up your thighs. Put your hand on your stomach and feel your abdominal muscles tighten. At the same time, your back is supported by the floor.

Lower Slowly lower your head and shoulder to the floor. Repeat the Slide and Lower through a phrase of music.

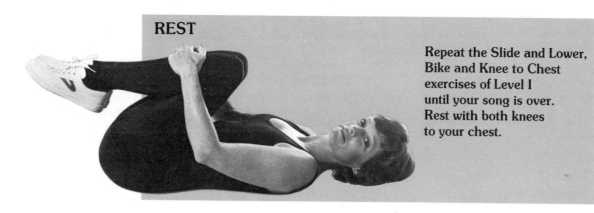

REST

Repeat the Slide and Lower, Bike and Knee to Chest exercises of Level I until your song is over. Rest with both knees to your chest.

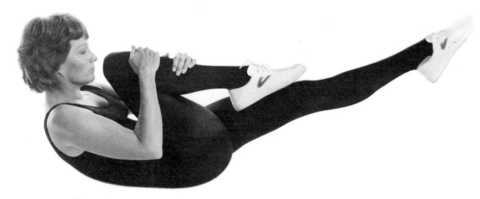

Bike Contract your abdominal muscles and pull your nose to your knee, extending your leg to the opposite wall in a bicycling movement. You are really working your abdominal muscles and your back is fully supported.

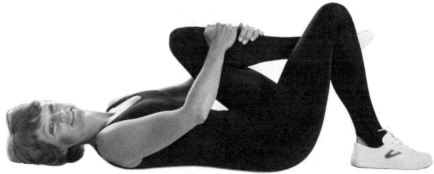

Knee to Chest Clasp your shins alternately, pulling the right and left knee to your chest.

LEVEL II SIT-UP

If you are comfortable with Level I,
and feel no back strain,
you are ready for Level II.

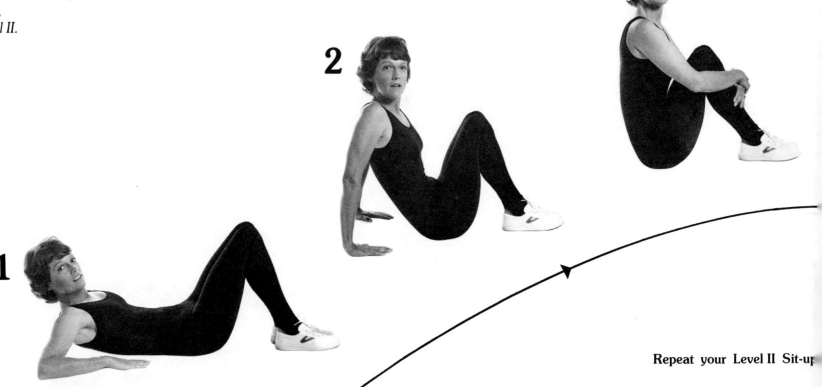

3

2

1

Repeat your Level II Sit-up

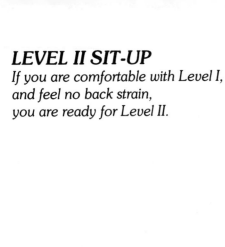

STARTING POSITION

Lying on your back, knees bent, feet flat, put your hands alongside your body under your armpits, palms down.

1 *Hands-down Roll-up*
Put your chin on your chest, round your back and shoulders, and roll up into a sit-up.

2 Use your hands to give you the added support you may need as you sit up. Think about your abdominal muscles and make them work for you.

3 Sit up tall with a straight back, hands clasping your knees.

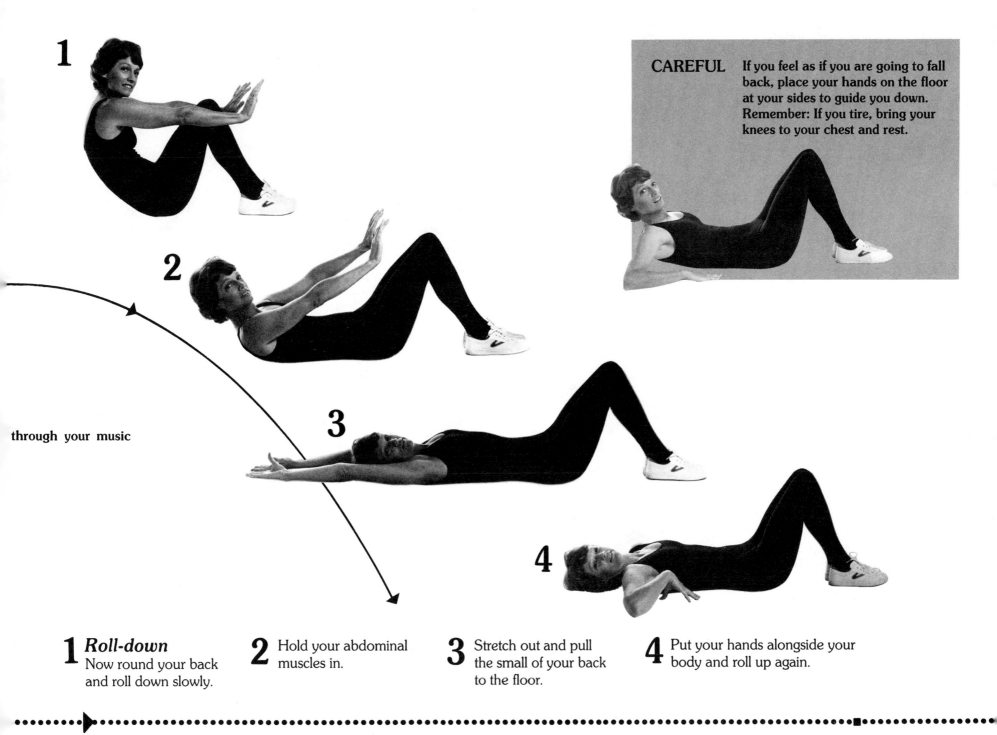

1

CAREFUL If you feel as if you are going to fall back, place your hands on the floor at your sides to guide you down. Remember: If you tire, bring your knees to your chest and rest.

2

through your music

3

4

1 *Roll-down*
Now round your back and roll down slowly.

2 Hold your abdominal muscles in.

3 Stretch out and pull the small of your back to the floor.

4 Put your hands alongside your body and roll up again.

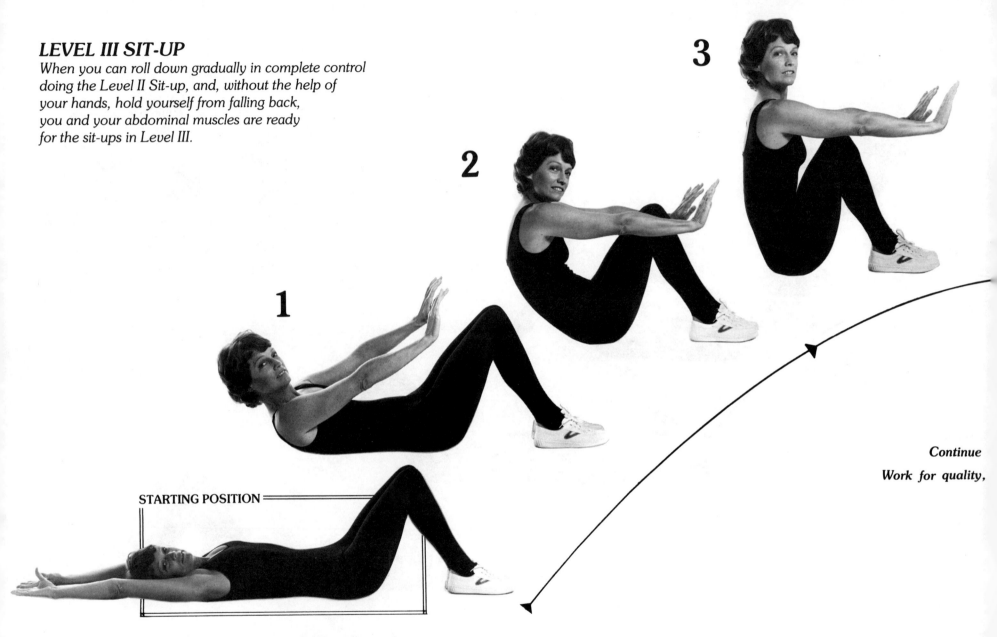

LEVEL III SIT-UP

When you can roll down gradually in complete control doing the Level II Sit-up, and, without the help of your hands, hold yourself from falling back, you and your abdominal muscles are ready for the sit-ups in Level III.

1

2

3

STARTING POSITION

Continue

Work for quality,

Stretch your arms overhead, abdominal muscles in and the small of your back tight to the floor.

1 *Hands-up Roll-up*
Contract your abdominal muscles, round your back, bring your arms forward and roll your back off the floor.

2 As you roll up, concentrate on your abdominal muscles. If your feet come off the floor or you must throw yourself to get up, you are straining your back. Return to Level II until your strength improves.

3 Sit tall.

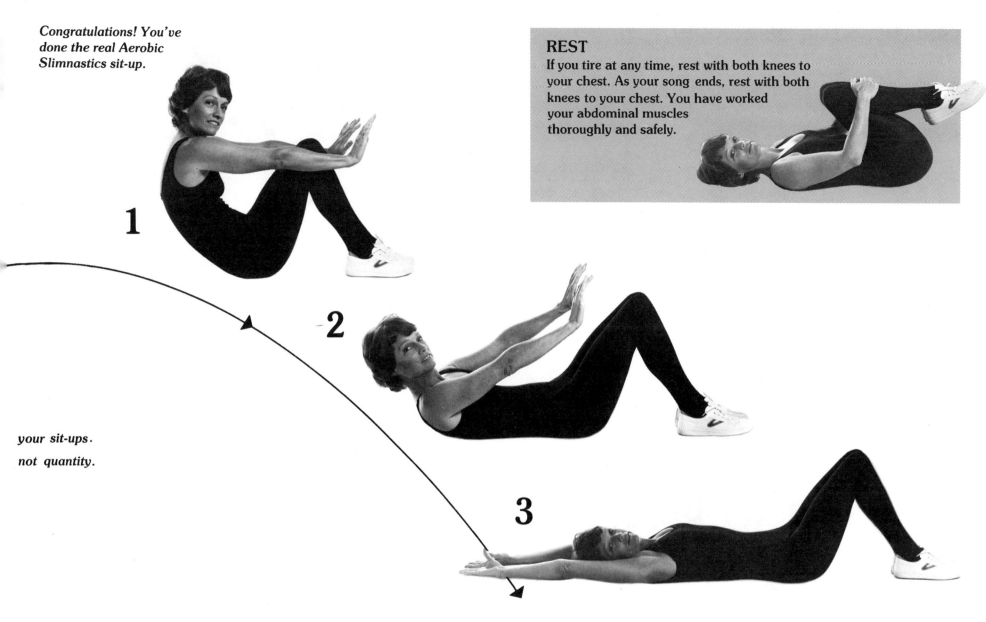

Congratulations! You've done the real Aerobic Slimnastics sit-up.

1

2

your sit-ups.

not quantity.

3

1 **Roll-down**
To roll back down, round your back and ease down gradually.

2 Concentrate on the lowering movement, making it smooth and controlled. The sit-up movement will come as your strength improves.

3 Before repeating your sit-up, stretch out, pull your abdominal muscles in, and flatten the small of your back to the floor.

VARIATIONS FOR THE FUN OF IT

*At Level II or Level III you can work
in some helpful variations.*

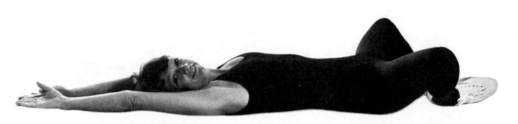

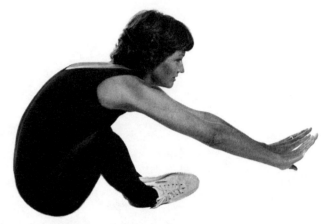

1 ***Wave*** Stretch your arms overhead. Bend your knees and drop them out to the side.

2 Roll up into a sit-up, keeping your knees apart. Push through your parted knees like a wave rolling onto a beach. *Really stretch . . .*

■ **Continue with Swing.**

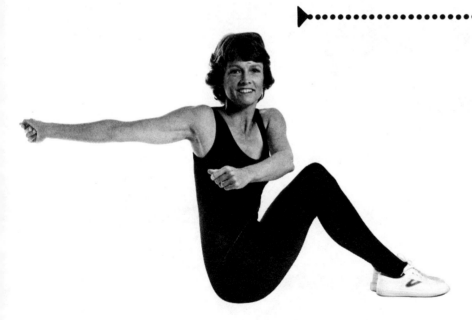

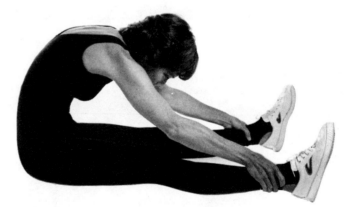

Swing At the top of your sit-up, before you roll down, swing to the right and left.

Stretch When you sit up, straighten your legs out in front of you and stretch your upper body to them.

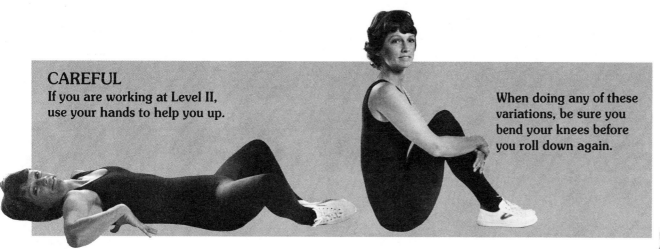

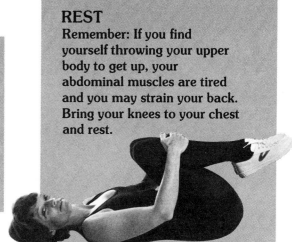

CAREFUL
If you are working at Level II, use your hands to help you up.

When doing any of these variations, be sure you bend your knees before you roll down again.

REST
Remember: If you find yourself throwing your upper body to get up, your abdominal muscles are tired and you may strain your back. Bring your knees to your chest and rest.

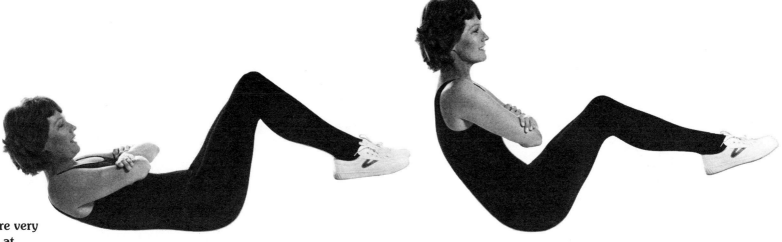

When you are very comfortable at Level III you may add the Advanced Sit-up. Mix it with sit-ups from Level III and Variations.

ADVANCED 1 *SIT-UP*
With knees well bent, lift your feet a few inches off the floor.

2 Contract your abdominal muscles and raise your upper back off the floor at the same time. Hold as long as you can, and then lower your legs and upper body simultaneously and carefully, always in full control.

◆ADVANCED■

Cool-down Stretch

Cooling-down routines are very important for your overall fitness well-being. These exercises will increase your flexibility and help prevent muscle soreness.

1 **Seated Stretch I**
Legs comfortably apart, stretch and bring your nose down to your right knee.

2 Sit up tall and reach high.

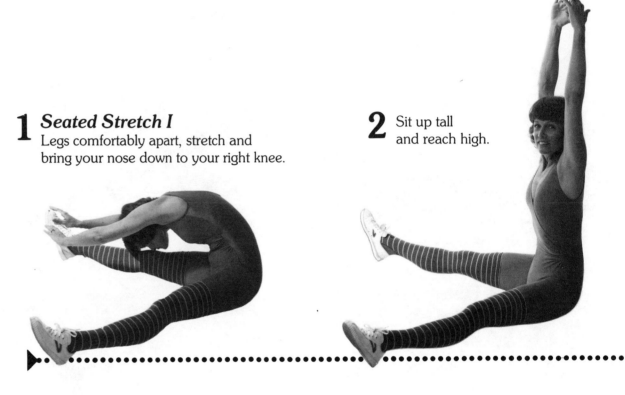

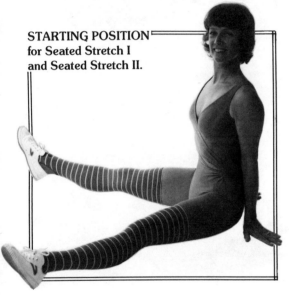

STARTING POSITION for Seated Stretch I and Seated Stretch II.

Sit up tall, legs comfortably apart, out in front of you. Straightening your lower back, lift your rib cage up off your waist.

1 **Seated Stretch II**
Pull your right ear to your right knee.

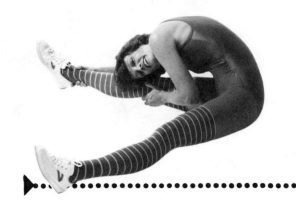

3 Stretch down to your left knee.

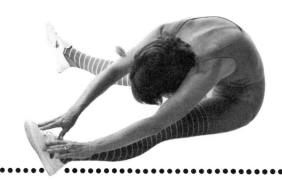

4 Sit up tall. Repeat, stretching nose to knee through several phrases of music.

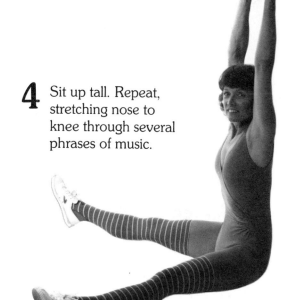

The music should remind you of a quiet, shady pond.
Suggestions:

1. "Lay Down Beside Me," Don Williams, *Expressions,* MCA Records
2. "Looks Like We Made It," Barry Manilow, *Greatest Hits,* Arista Records
3. "Sweet Survivor," Peter, Paul & Mary, *Reunion,* Warner Brothers Records

■ **Move back to your starting position and continue with Seated Stretch II.**

2 Sit up tall.

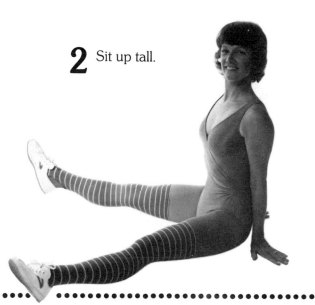

3 Pull your left ear to your left knee. Let your arms do the work.

4 Sit up tall and repeat these stretches to your music.

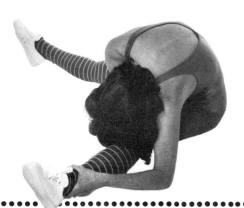

A daruma is a Japanese folk doll—roly and round on the bottom. No matter how the doll rolls to one side or the other, it always rights itself.

1 **Daruma Stretch**
Fold your feet in tight to your body. Knees out to the sides. Sit up tall.

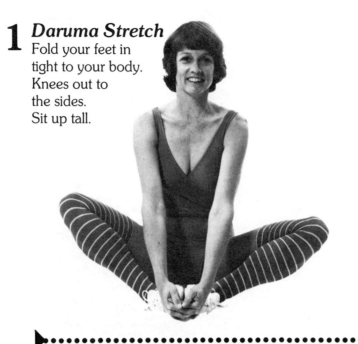

2 Round your back and pull your nose toward your feet. Sit up tall again.

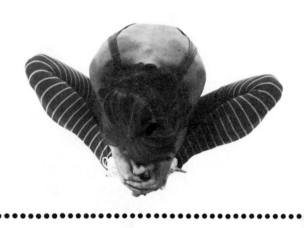

1 **Bounce, Stretch, and Lift**
Sitting tall with your legs extended in front of you, bounce your right foot once over your left leg. Return to starting position and . . .

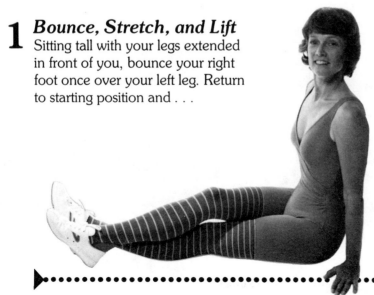

2 . . . bounce your left foot once over your right leg.

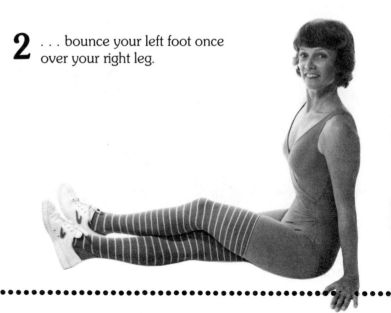

3 Tighten your buttocks, and rock from side to side.

Think about the round-bottomed daruma and roll to your music.

This exercise will feel so good! Repeat with your music.

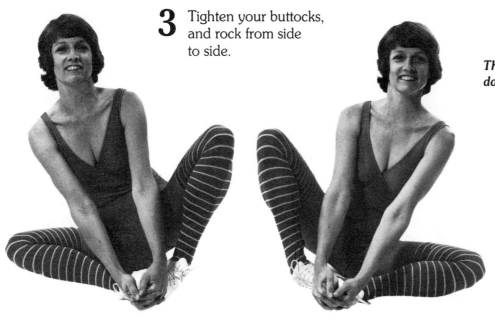

■ Move on to **Bounce, Stretch, and Lift.**

3 Stretch your nose to your knee.

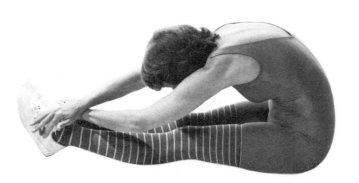

4 Put your hands behind you and lift your body off the floor.

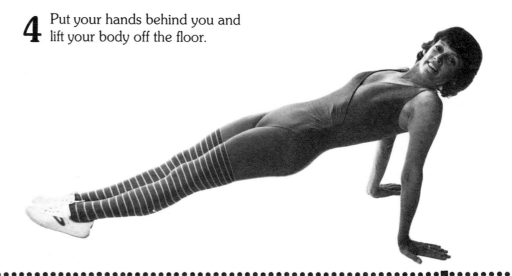

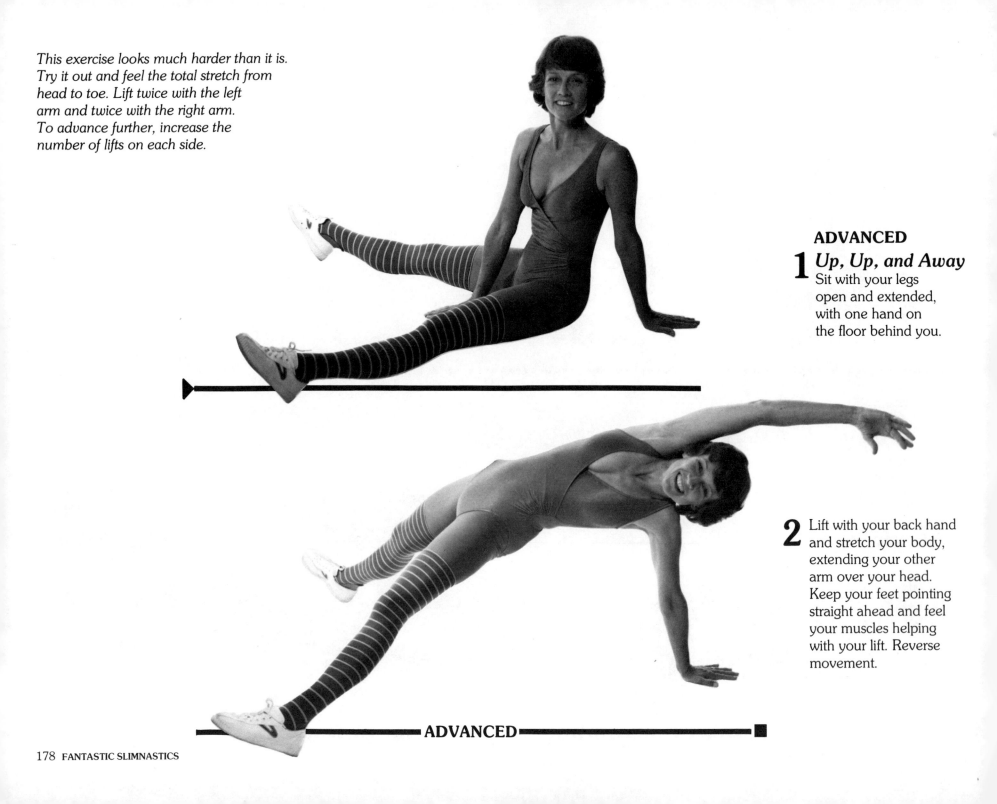

This exercise looks much harder than it is. Try it out and feel the total stretch from head to toe. Lift twice with the left arm and twice with the right arm. To advance further, increase the number of lifts on each side.

ADVANCED

1 *Up, Up, and Away*
Sit with your legs open and extended, with one hand on the floor behind you.

2 Lift with your back hand and stretch your body, extending your other arm over your head. Keep your feet pointing straight ahead and feel your muscles helping with your lift. Reverse movement.

ADVANCED

GOOD HEALTH AND GOOD SEX

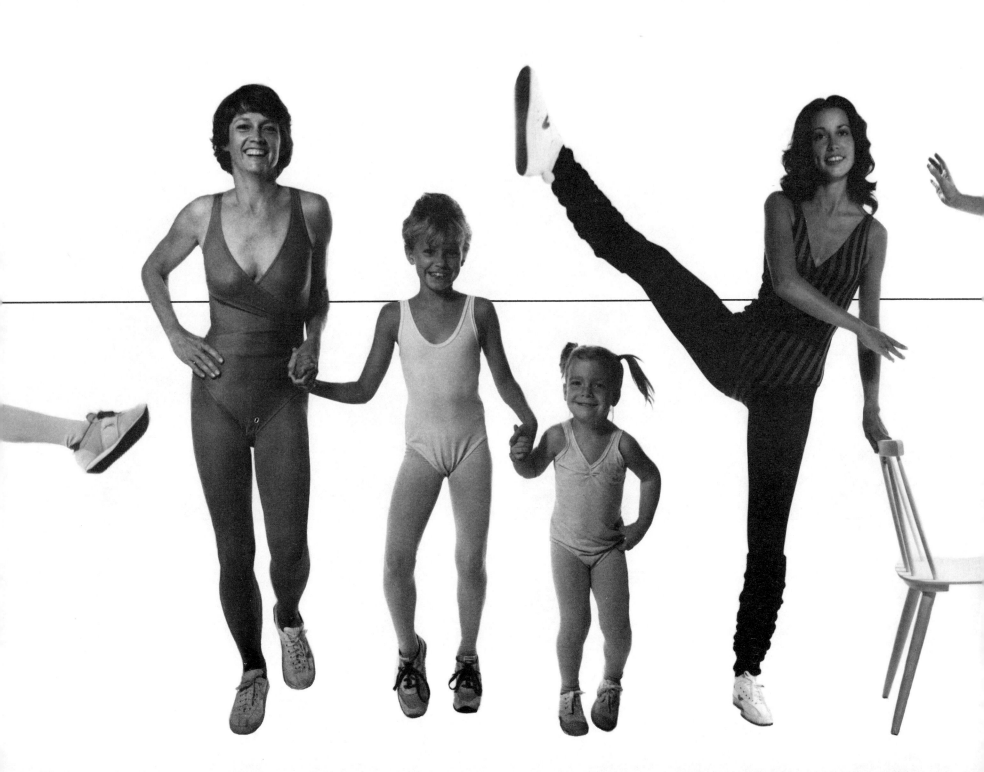

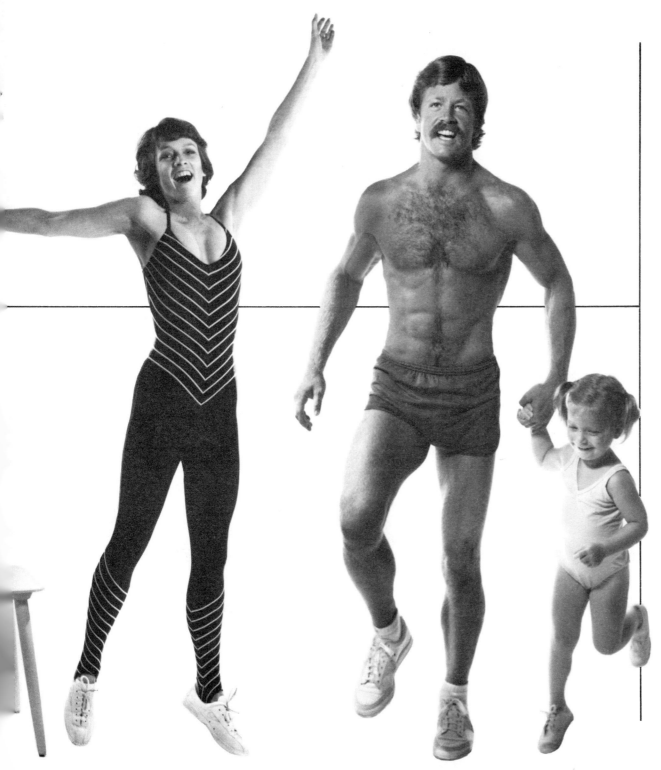

CONTENTS

Sexercises

Here it is. Sexercise will:

- *strengthen your lower back*
- *stop urinary incontinence*
- *firm your abdominal muscles and shape your buttocks and thighs*
- *improve your sex life*

These exercises strengthen the muscles that hold you up, inside and out. For all of us, this may be the most important chapter in the book.

Sexercises

Strengthen the muscles of your buttocks, lower back, abdominal muscles, and the pelvic muscles in between.

For men and women alike, strong pelvic muscles will hold your internal organs in place. When your pelvic floor is firm and strong, and everything inside of you is where it should be, your life will be more comfortable.

The music should remind you of a warm moonlit evening.

Suggestions:

1. "Waking Up Alone," Paul Williams, *Just an Old-Fashioned Love Song,* A & M Records
2. "Blues for Lauren-Marie," Roger Whittaker, *The Magical World of Roger Whittaker,* Victor Records
3. "Canon in D," Jean-François Paillard Chamber Orchestra, RCA Records

1 *Prone Pelvic Push*
Lie prone on the floor, resting your head on your hands.

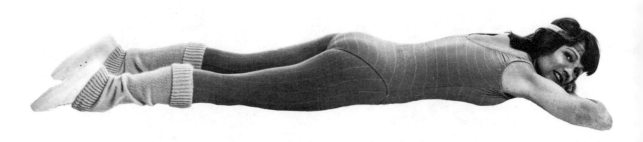

1 *Bridge* Roll over and lie on your back, with your knees bent and your feet flat on the floor. Gently arch the small of your back, making a little bridge.

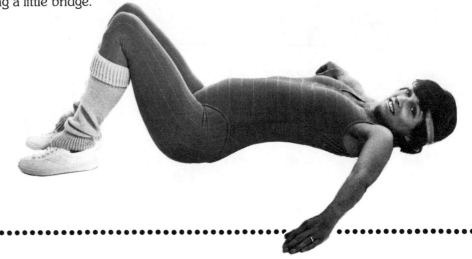

2 Pull your buttocks together. Pull your abdominal muscles in and tuck your pelvis back. Your pubic bone will be tight to the floor. Hold and tighten every muscle. The arch in the small of your back will flatten out. Hold through a phrase of music. Then really relax all your muscles. Try tucking under gradually to a count of five. Relax out to a count of five.

These exercises are so easy to do.

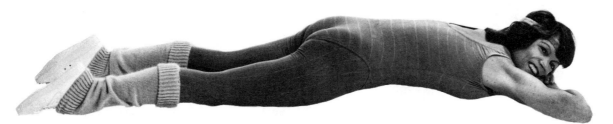

■ Move on
to Bridge.

2 Collapse the bridge by pushing the small of your back to the floor. Pinch your buttocks together, hold your abdominal muscles in, and tighten everything you can inside of you. H-O-L-D and then relax.

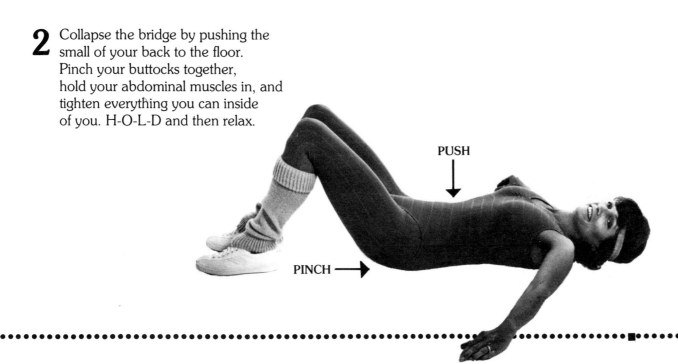

PUSH

PINCH →

Ski Slope Lift your pelvis off the floor, making a smooth ski slope with your body. Without arching your back, tighten your buttocks, your abdominal muscles, and your pelvic muscles, inside and out. Hold as if you are holding a quarter between your buttocks and it must not fall out. When you get very good, pretend you have a dime.

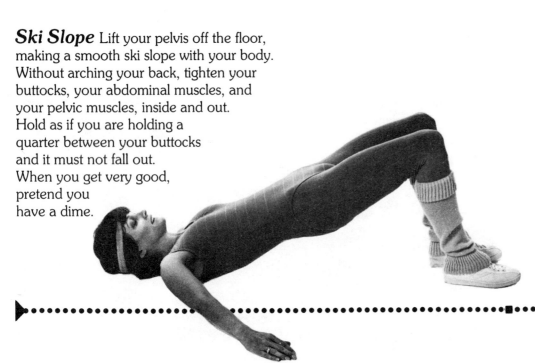

1 Knee to Chest Round your back and gradually roll down from the Ski Slope position. Put your hands on your shins and hug your right knee to your chest . . .

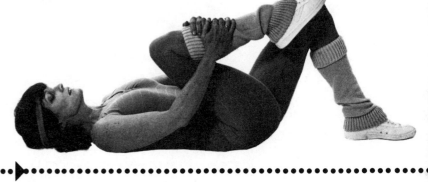

1 Easy Roll-over Lie on your back, hugging your knees to your chest. Roll to one side.

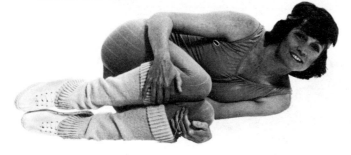

2 Keeping your knees in . . .

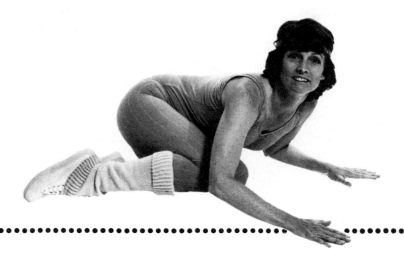

2 . . . your left knee . . .

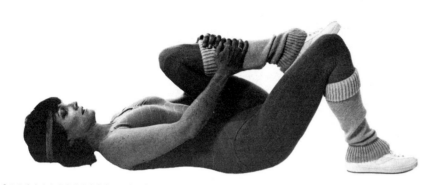

3 . . . and then hug both of your knees to your chest. Feel the muscles in your lower back relax.

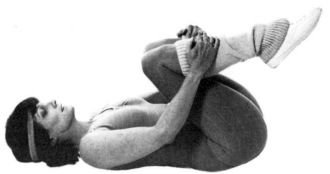

■ Move on to Easy Roll-over.

Repeat Easy Roll-over on the other side.

3 . . . ease up gradually . . .

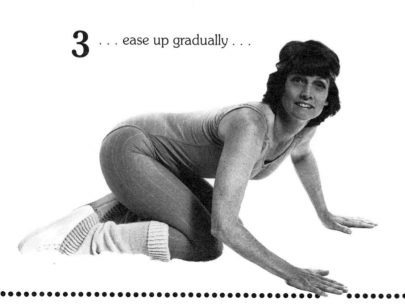

4 . . . to all fours.

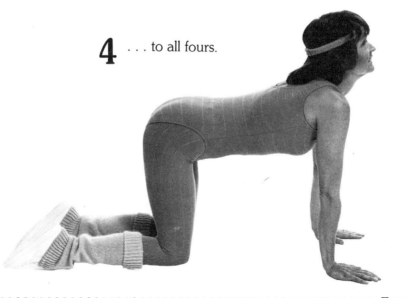

Angry Cat On all fours, round your back like a Halloween cat. Pull your abdominal muscles in, pull your buttocks together, and hold tight with all the muscles inside of you.

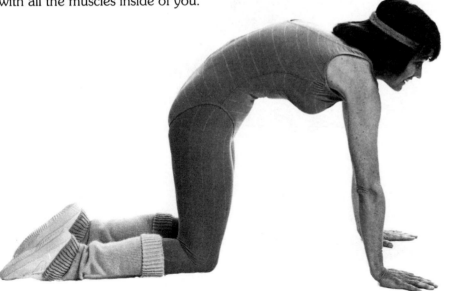

Tired Horse Gently drop your back like a Tired Horse, lifting your chin and keeping your elbows straight. Repeat several times.

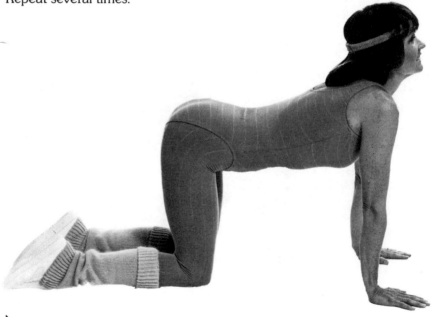

Congratulations! You have completed your Aerobic Slimnastics class. That's all of it—the hard work and the fun. We did it together, and you did it for yourself. How do you feel? You're on your way to being trimmer, slimmer, and stronger. Have a drink of water and a refreshing shower. Let's have a class again tomorrow. If not tomorrow, then we have a definite date for the next day. Meanwhile, step back into your life and enjoy yourself.

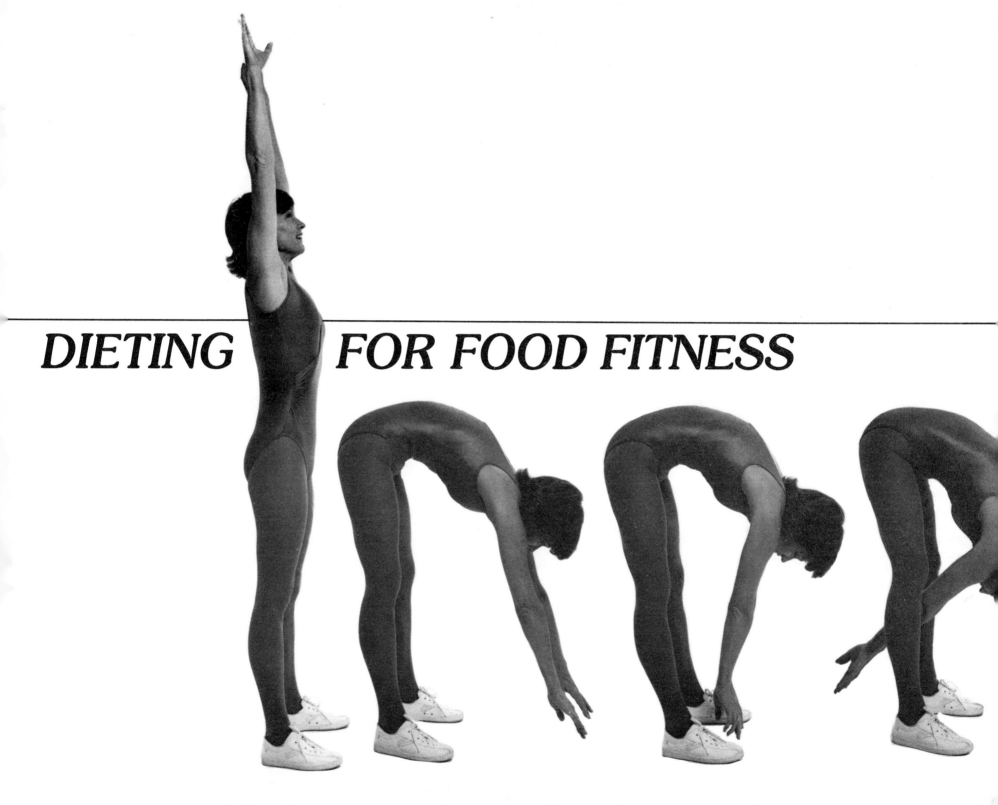

DIETING FOR FOOD FITNESS

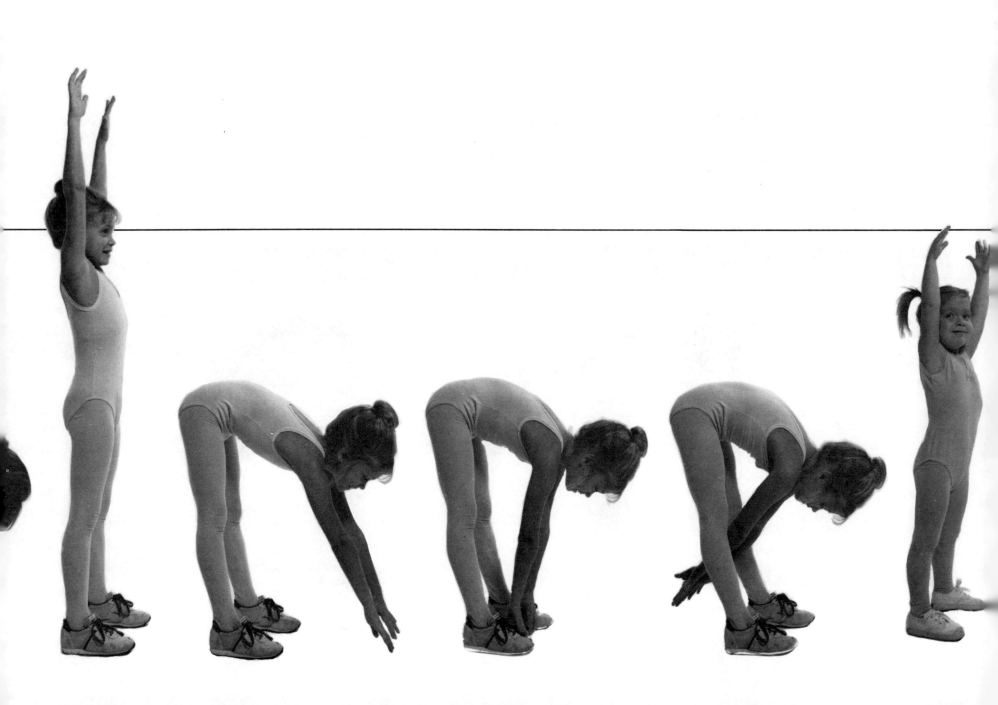

Hooked on Health

Don't stop now!

Fitness is a whole way of life. Looking and feeling our best is what we're all after, and Aerobic Slimnastics offers a sensible, simple way to make the most out of living. There are two ingredients in this program—aerobic exercise and a well-balanced diet emphasizing fresh foods. Sounds easy, doesn't it?

Exercise is the main variable in estimating adult energy needs. Aerobic workouts are high calorie burners—you burn three hundred to five hundred calories during an Aerobic Slimnastics session, and your metabolic rate will remain higher than normal for about six hours after the workout. This is so comforting when you go to your desk after early morning exercise—you are actually burning more calories through the morning than you would had you skipped your exercise session to read the paper.

Maybe you're thinking, "If I exercise, I'll eat more." Not so, according to medical studies. You feel hungry when your blood sugar level drops. When you exercise regularly, your blood sugar level stabilizes. You may actually eat less. When you exercise, the large muscles need more blood and oxygen. Less blood and oxygen are delivered to the stomach, which decreases sensations of hunger. After exercise, food passes through your digestive tract more quickly than it would otherwise, so you actually absorb fewer calories. Athletes report a meal can pass through their systems in as little as four to eight hours whereas sedentary people need twelve to twenty-four hours to digest a meal fully. Combining this phys-

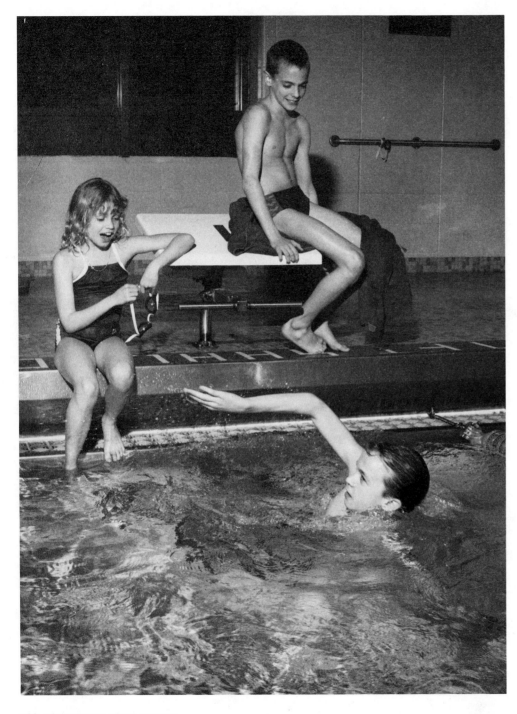

Physical fitness is a way of life for my children.

ical tendency with an improved high-fiber diet increases bowel health, which has positive implications for a range of problems from constipation to cancer.

Once exercise becomes a part of your life, weight loss will follow naturally as you seek out the amounts and kinds of food that will enhance your fitness. Regular exercise provides a sense of discipline that extends into other areas of your life, and you gain a new sense of commitment that makes other life changes somehow seem easier. Exercise will put you in touch with your body. You'll know what feels good and what doesn't. You'll recognize the sugar blues and the effects of too much salt or junk food. Your body will crave fresh fruits and vegetables to replace lost fluids and minerals. I call this phenomenon Food Fitness.

My own family's Food Fitness evolved through exercise. All three of my children spend up to two hours daily swimming. For the first time in years, I can throw away half of stale birthday cakes, and cookies remain unopened. With one teenager and two preteens in the house, I know this seems unbelievable. But I find that the foods that everyone loves are nuts, seeds, fresh and dried fruits, and fruit juices.

Together with exercise, a well-balanced diet emphasizing fresh foods is the second necessary ingredient for total fitness. Fresh foods will keep you away from the nutritionally empty salted and sugared processed foods that beckon to you from TV commercials and the grocer's shelf. Instead of feeling deprived while dieting, you will get special flavors from fresh ingredients that will make each meal seem unique.

In our busy lives, opening a can or a frozen

dinner often seems quicker and more appealing than sticking with freshness, even though it takes just minutes to slice crisp florets from a head of cauliflower or broccoli, steam them until the color intensifies, and present them on the table. I think the problem may lie in our perception of fresh vegetables as presented by the fine chefs of the world. Fresh carrots look beautiful curled and julienned, but those same carrots taste fine simply sliced. French-cut green beans are wonderful, to be sure, but the flavor is just as outstanding when the beans are chopped. Whenever recipes called for peeled tomatoes, I was intimidated by the thought of removing that slippery fruit from its casing. But I soon discovered chopped tomatoes are delicious and fresh-tasting, skin and all! The joy of stir-frying or steam cooking is that there is one pot for everything.

My family has been very helpful in freshening up our diet. Kevin mashes the potatoes with enthusiasm while Robbie likes to flex his muscles with the apple sauce grinder. Dana makes the popcorn. Everyone is intrigued by the sprouter and yogurt maker.

I introduced these changes to my family gradually and quietly. Understanding the pressure of advertising and peers, I never said, no, you absolutely can't have something. Instead, we discussed the benefits of a well-balanced diet and fresh foods and our kitchen was open to taste-testing. Conversation was stimulated by some excellent charts posted on the side of our refrigerator that explain additives and nutritional content. (You can send away for these charts. The address is listed on page 207.)

I discovered that children love to read labels. It was primarily this activity that banished the sugared cereals from our kitchen. Picture my oldest child seated at the breakfast table reciting the ingredients of one of the children's presweetened cereals, "sugar, brown sugar, Mono and Diglycerides, FD&C Red No. 3, FD&C Yellow No. 5, FD&C Yellow No. 6, BHA, FD&C Blue No. 2, FD&C Green, No. 3 . . ." as our faces turned green.

All of our discussions served to educate the family and reinforce the commitment I've made to myself and to them with Food Fitness. We've learned the importance of a balanced diet, the necessity of vitamins and minerals, and the problems of too much sugar and salt. Let's look together at good nutrition and the way to a healthier you.

Balancing Your Diet

CARBOHYDRATES

If you believed all the TV commercials touting the quick pick-me-up effect of candy bars and soft drinks, you would think processed sugar was the answer to all our energy needs. That's not the case. Glycogen, a sugar converted from the food you eat, is what gives your body "get-up and go." Complex carbohydrates such as fruits, vegetables, grains, nuts, and seeds are the best sources of this body fuel.

Unlike simple sugars, complex carbohydrates do not scramble your system. In addition to providing important vitamins and minerals, these efficient energy sources are easily broken down into glucose and stored for energy.

There's more! Complex carbohydrates are also excellent sources of fiber. Since fiber is undigestible, it adds no calories as it passes through your system, absorbing water and keeping your bowels healthy. Fiber also absorbs bile salts and cholesterol, lowering your cholesterol level.

Active people must rely heavily on carbohydrates for energy. I recommend a daily diet of 50 to 65 percent carbohydrates. With Aerobic Slimnastics, you will be active enough to utilize this vital energy source without putting on excess fat.

FATS

What about fat in our diet? Fat is classified as saturated or unsaturated. Saturated fats come from animals and have been found to contribute to heart disease. Unsaturated fats are found in plants. Studies of primarily meat-eating and primarily vegetable-eating societies indicate that the latter have a better health record. In today's average American diet, fats and oils provide 40 to 45 percent of the day's calories—more than double that of our ancestors' diets two hundred years ago. This dietary trend has been accompanied by a perplexing increase in obesity, diabetes, gall bladder disease, breast and bowel cancer, and heart attacks.

A small amount of fat is necessary to insulate and protect the body and provide a medium for fat-soluble vitamins. In marathon athletic events, the fat stored in the muscles of the endurance athlete gives him or her a source of energy after the muscles have exhausted their glycogen supply.

Ideally, a woman's body weight is 18 to 22 percent fat whereas a man's is 12 to 15 percent. It is just this difference in fat storage that may give women athletes the edge over men in marathon events. Who can forget the fresh-faced exhilaration of 1981 and 1982 New York marathoner Grete Waitz as she crossed the finish line, looking as if she might be ready for another few miles.

Since most of us are not marathon athletes, however, we should eat fat sparingly. The bare facts are that the calories in fats will make you fat. Fats should make up no more than 20 to 30 percent of your daily diet if you are aiming for ideal body weight. Beyond that level, you will store fat, making your heart work harder with each extra pound of body baggage.

PROTEINS

Protein is the primary building material for your cells and tissue. It is essential for healthy red blood cells and the production of enzymes, hormones, and antibodies. Protein contains twenty-two amino acids, the body's building blocks. Since your body can manufacture only fourteen amino acids, you must obtain the remaining eight from your diet.

Good sources of animal protein include meat, fish, poultry, eggs, cheese, and milk, whereas nuts, beans, peas, seeds, and whole grains are good sources of plant protein. Animal proteins provide all eight of the amino acids you need, but unfortunately also contain a lot of fat and cholesterol. Although plant proteins are incomplete, combining your vegetables will fulfill nutritional needs. Eating a small amount of high-quality animal protein such as chicken and fish or mixing plant proteins are your best health bets. Plant protein combinations, such as whole grains and legumes or seeds and legumes, are most effective when you eat them at the same meal.

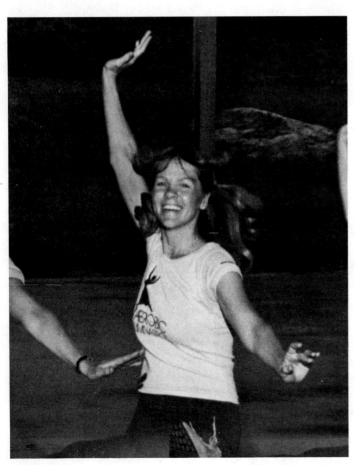

"I love the whole experience. This is saving my life."

Contrary to the old coach's tale calling for steak before the big game, protein is not a good source of immediate energy and must be converted into a carbohydrate before it can be utilized by your body. Toxic by-products of this conversion process must be excreted, causing a strain on your kidneys. This lengthy digestive process ties up blood and oxygen sorely needed by your heart and active muscles.

High protein-low carbohydrate fad diets can wreak considerable havoc on your body. Without carbohydrates, your body is forced to use protein for energy, limiting cell repair, breaking down muscle tissue, and overworking the kidneys. Students of mine on these diets have complained of nausea, constipation, dizziness, headaches, fatigue, bad breath, and body odor. High protein-low carbohydrate diets, all-fruit diets, and fasting are among the regimens that can actually do your body more harm than good. Why do these fad diets survive?

Initially, the fad diet produces weight loss, a situation that puts a smile on the face of any dieter. But is this weight loss fat? The digestion of fats and proteins in these diets produces toxic wastes that are removed with water through urination. Generally, weight loss is, in fact, water loss and, if the diet is continued, muscle loss. If you go off the fad diet and start consuming more calories than you burn, you may be worse off than when you started, since you will replace the water and gain back fat instead of muscle.

If the average American diet of meats, fats, processed foods, sugar, and salt is creating health problems and making us fat, what kind of diet is best? A diet that contains a good nutritional balance of carbohydrates, fats, proteins, vitamins, and minerals each day in quantities equal to (not more or less than) your body's energy requirements. But how much should you eat? Probably less, considering the fact that our nation's number-one nutritional problem is obesity. You need energy—that is, calories—but from birth to old age your energy requirements decline continuously. It has been proposed that energy allowances for people over fifty be reduced to 90 percent of the amount required as a young adult. Consequently, as you get older, you require fewer and fewer calories.

The following chart shows the approximate number of calories women need each day to maintain their present weight. Men will need more calories. Note that the number of calories varies according to your activity level. The calories required for minimal activity are considered a maintenance figure for most people. It is the number of calories it takes to keep your body functioning day to day if your life is as sedentary as the average American's tends to be. A person who exercises regularly and strenuously is considered moderately active, and someone like a professional dancer or athlete is considered highly active.

CALORIES REQUIRED TO MAINTAIN YOUR PRESENT WEIGHT				
WEIGHT	INACTIVE	MINIMALLY ACTIVE	MODERATELY ACTIVE	HIGHLY ACTIVE
	12 cal. per lb. of body wt.	15 cal per lb. of body wt.	17 cal. per lb. of body wt.	20+ cal per lb. of body wt.
100	1200	1500	1700	2000
110	1320	1650	1870	2200
120	1440	1800	2040	2400
130	1560	1950	2210	2600
140	1680	2100	2380	2800
150	1800	2250	2550	3000
160	1920	2400	2720	3200
170	2040	2550	2890	3400
180	2160	2700	3060	3600

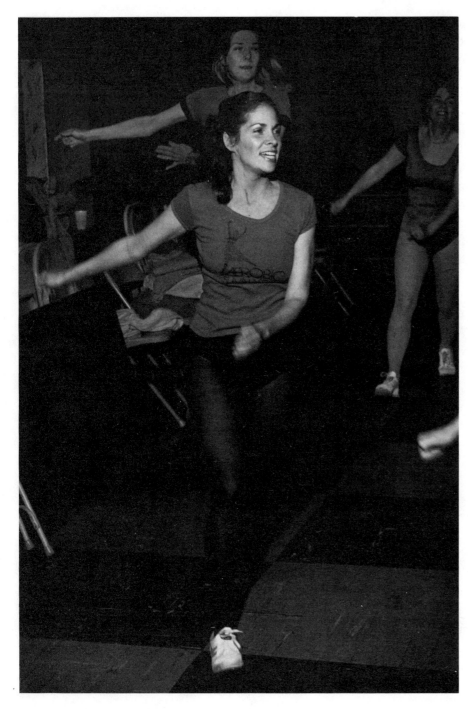

"I can't begin to share with you how much Aerobic Slimnastics has changed me, not only physically, but intellectually, emotionally, and spiritually."

To calculate the number of calories it takes to maintain your present weight, use the following formula:

Weight × the number = the number of
of calories/ calories per day
pound in needed to maintain
your activity your present weight
level

If you exercise aerobically three times a week, you should consider yourself in the moderately active category and should calculate 17 calories per pound of body weight to maintain your present weight.

If you are overweight and want to lose, calories do count! All diets are based on them in one way or another. You must lose the surplus calories stored as fat. There are no miracle diets. Current scientific evidence points to only one way to lose weight: taking in fewer calories in food than you use up in energy. One pound of body fat equals 3,500 calories. To lose one pound a week, you must eat 500 calories less than your body uses up for seven days. In other words, 7 days × 500 calories = 3,500 calories or one pound of body fat.

Now figure out how many calories you need to maintain your present weight and subtract 500 from this number to see how many calories you should eat per day in order to lose one pound per week. A pound per week may not sound like much, but this is a lifetime eating plan. To make this plan work like a diet for you, you'll need a kitchen scale that will help you learn portion sizes, and a good book on the caloric content of foods. To keep this plan nutritionally sound, it should include each day:

4 to 6 ounces of protein:
   meat, fish, poultry, eggs, dairy products
1 citrus fruit
1 serving dark green or deep yellow vegetable
1 serving bread or cereal
8 ounces milk
6 to 8 eight-ounce glasses of water.

This is a reasonable and livable way to maintain your weight while caring for your body.

SUGAR

Picture 13 ten-pound boxes of sugar stacked on top of one another. That's the amount of sugar the average American consumes each year. The vision makes my teeth hurt and my stomachache. "How can that possibly be?" you ask. "I don't ever put sugar on my cereal." Sugar, like salt, has become an invisible ingredient in many processed foods. Since the government requires package listing of ingredients by amounts, food manufacturers can hide the sugar content, placing it lower in the list, by breaking it down into smaller amounts of raw or brown sugar, honey, molasses, corn syrup, fructose, dextrose, maltose, and glucose. But put it all together and it spells SUGAR and is among the top three ingredients in such diverse items as nondairy creamers, catsup, and gelatin desserts.

Sugar's role in tooth decay gets a lot of press. But did you know that sugar also raises the level of cholesterol and fats in the blood, and is thus one of the "bad guys" in obesity, arteriosclerosis, heart attacks, and strokes? It is also linked to kidney stones, allergies, diabetes (high blood sugar), and hypoglycemia (low blood sugar). Sugar increases stomach acidity, contributes to dehydration, interferes with cell respiration, and uses up vital potassium and magnesium.

Simple sugar actually increases hunger. It is full of empty calories and devoid of minerals and nutrients. When you eat that tempting piece of chocolate cake, your blood sugar level immediately rises. In response, your body produces the hormone insulin. Insulin gobbles up the sugar from the cake and then some, causing a precipitous drop in your blood sugar level. Then you feel hungry and down, so you crave more sugar to pep you up, and the roller coaster ride begins again. The more sugar you have, the more your body will want and you can become addicted to sugar.

If you need a sweetener when cooking, substitute small amounts of honey, pure maple sugar, or blackstrap molasses. Eat a piece of fruit if you crave something sweet. Fruit contains fiber that slows down the breakdown of sugar and helps you avoid the highs and lows associated with processed sugar. Free yourself of the sugar habit by gradually, patiently, and conscientiously cutting it out of your diet over time.

MINERALS

Your body is a gold mine of valuable minerals. There are six minerals that the body needs in large amounts and at least fourteen trace minerals. Minerals regulate vital body functions such as muscle contractions, nerve impulses, and body-water storage. Keep in mind that chemical additives, preservatives, food processing, and lengthy storage play havoc with minerals. For the important minerals so essential to good health, turn to the foods that come from the earth—the vegetables, fruits, nuts, and grains that will brighten up your daily diet. Buy healthy-looking produce. Remember, freshness is the key! Four minerals—potassium, calcium, magnesium, and sodium—are of particular interest to the exercising person.

Potassium

Potassium keeps your body from overheating. Working muscles release potassium into your bloodstream, increasing the flow of blood, widening the blood vessels, and carrying heat away from your muscles. Its job done, potassium is carried away from your body in sweat and urine. Potassium deficiency causes muscle weakness, cramping, crankiness, and overall fatigue. Unfortunately, your body doesn't have a potassium depletion warning signal like the thirst that signals dehydration. Natural diuretics and diuretic medication, including the medicine given for premenstrual tension, wash vital mineral-filled water from your body. Heavy perspiration, chronic diarrhea, and excessive salt intake can lead to potassium deficiency. Although cramps can be caused by a muscle injury, most of the cramping I see in Aerobic Slimnastics classes or hear about from students is the result of a deficiency in minerals, particularly potassium. Muscle cramps are painful contractions of muscle fiber. For immediate relief, massage the area and try to stretch and squeeze your muscle. For those nightmarish calf or toe cramps that wake you with a start, flex and point your foot and massage the affected area. For long-term relief, increase your intake of mineral-rich fruits and vegetables. I have seen positive results from cramp sufferers who followed this advice: A banana a day keeps muscle cramps away. Fruits, vegetables, nuts, soybeans, wheat germ, rye flour, and molasses are all rich in potassium.

Calcium

Calcium is vital for strong bones and teeth, and healthy muscles, nerves, and blood. If your body does not have enough calcium to service the muscles, it will immediately steal it from your bones. Together with potassium, calcium helps allay muscle cramps, including premenstrual cramps.

Fortunately, almost no calcium is lost through sweat and urine. In fact, exercise has been found to increase calcium absorption and decrease calcium loss from bones.

The dairy products, milk, cheese, and yogurt are all rich in calcium and vitamin D. Sardines and salmon (with bones), green leafy vegetables, asparagus, beans, nuts, egg yolks, and tofu are also fine sources of this essential mineral.

Magnesium

Magnesium controls muscle contractions and appears to be a natural tranquilizer, soothing nerves as well as muscles. This mineral is an essential part of many enzymes and is also necessary for digestion of proteins. A shortage of magnesium will make you tired and weak and will contribute to tense, twitching muscles.

Foods rich in magnesium are green leafy vegetables, nuts, corn, beans, rice oatmeal, dark breads, and beer.

Sodium

The sodium in salt is essential to life. Two thirds of your body is filled with a salty solution, your kidneys maintaining the delicate balance of salt to water in this internal sea. This balance affects the vital functions of the heart and nerves. If your body loses too much salt and the balance is tipped, you may dehydrate, develop muscle cramps, and become vulnerable to heat stroke. But, paradoxically, sodium has its hazardous side, which has recently caused it to receive mixed reviews from the health experts. Too much salt in your blood can cause fluid retention, aggravating premenstrual swelling. Salt in higher doses can drive fluids and important minerals from the body, forcing the heart and kidneys to work overtime. Too much salt is also a factor in high blood pressure. Given these dangers, salt boxes should be labeled like cigarette packages: "The contents are potentially hazardous to your health." Americans consume an average of two and a half teaspoons of salt per day, far more than most need. Processed, canned, and baked goods are loaded with salt. Notice in the chart on opposite page how salt content increases with processing.

An overly salty diet and exercise do not go well together. If I have salty food before an Aerobic Slimnastics class, I struggle uphill all day to replace fluids and quench my thirst.

Our American diet provides adequate sodium for good health. Additional salt tips the balance. Take the salt out of your recipes. You will feel better and begin to appreciate your food. I have long felt that salt masks the natural flavor of foods and dulls the taste buds. Serve the freshest veg-etables slightly undercooked to preserve the flavor. Investigate fresh herbs. Imagine the delicate flavor of fresh mushrooms, eggplant, and juicy red tomatoes. Treat yourself to really fresh eggs and the subtle taste of salt-free butter. Take the salt shaker off the table and you will discover a world of subtle, natural, fresh flavors.

VITAMINS

The best way to obtain the vitamins you need is by eating a well-balanced diet. There is, however, a healthy debate among health professionals over just how much you need of certain vitamins, and from where you should get them. Your body also needs varying amount of vitamins at different stages of your life, further complicating the situation. Certain life-styles create countless circumstances leading to vitamin deficiency. You may need a vitamin supplement if you are exposed to smog, large doses of sun, or ultraviolet light. Excessive amounts of alcohol, coffee, sugar, and fast foods also drain your body's vitamin supply. If your life has been made stressful by illness, surgery, or medication, keep a watch for vitamin deficiency.

Each vitamin has a personality all its own.

A is for Active

Vitamin A is found in orange, yellow, and green fruits; vegetables such as carrots, sweet potatoes, tomatoes, and apricots; and also in beef, liver, and dairy products. This vitamin keeps your eyes healthy. The skin and mucous membranes of the throat, nasal passages, and bronchial tubes, and the vaginal and urinary tracts rely on vitamin A.

FRESH FOOD & PROCESSING = INCREASED SALT

APPLE 2	APPLESAUCE 1 cup 6	APPLE PIE ⅛ frozen 208			
BREAD 1 slice, white 114	POUND CAKE 1 slice 171	ENGLISH MUFFIN 293			
BUTTER 1 tbsp., unsalted 2	BUTTER 1 tbsp., salted 116	MARGARINE 1 tbsp. 140			
CHICKEN ½ breast 69	CHICKEN PIE frozen 907	CHICKEN DINNER fast food 2,243			
CORN 1	CORN FLAKES 1 cup 256	CANNED CORN 1 cup 384			
CUCUMBER 7 slices 2	CUCUMBER with salad dressing 234	DILL PICKLE 928			
GRAPES 10, seedless 1	GRAPE JELLY 1 tbsp. 3	WHITE WINE 4 oz. domestic 19			
LEMON 1	SOY SAUCE 1 tbsp. 1,029	SALT 1 tbsp. 1,938			
MILK 1 cup 122	DRY MILK ½ cup 322	COTTAGE CHEESE 4 oz. 457			
PORK 3 oz. 59	BACON 4 slices 548	HAM 3 oz. 1,114			
POTATO 5	POTATO CHIPS 10 200	INSTANT MASHED 1 cup 485			
STEAK 3 oz. 55	LARGE BURGER fast food 990	MEAT LOAF frozen dinner 1,304			
TOMATO 14	TOMATO SOUP 1 cup 932	TOMATO SAUCE 1 cup 1,498			
TUNA 3 oz. 50	CANNED TUNA 3 oz. 384	TUNA POT PIE frozen 715			
WATER 8 oz., tap 12	CLUB SODA 8 oz. 39	ANTACID in water 564			

Content in milligrams

Based on data from *Time*, March 1982.

B is for Building

The B's—thiamine, riboflavin, niacin, vitamin B_6, vitamin B_{12}, pantothenic acid, folacin, and biotin—are the nerve and energy vitamins. Fortunately, they are usually found together. Good sources for these vitamins include green leafy vegetables, whole grains, beans, nuts, seeds, dairy products, and liver.

Depression, irritability, poor concentration, paranoia, anxiety, and insomnia are frequently related to a deficiency in the B vitamins. Besides preventing a nervous breakdown, the B's help the body turn carbohydrates into glucose, which feeds the muscles and brain. The B's also protect your skin and aid in blood production.

Vitamins B_6 and B_{12} are of particular interest to women. Birth control pills often tax our B_{12} supply. Even a slight deficiency of B_{12} can cause fatigue and irritability. Animal products are rich in B_{12}, which is the reason vegetarians must watch their intake of this important vitamin. Some doctors claim B_6 may reduce premenstrual tension.

C is for Coping

Vitamin C is a wonderful antidote. It helps your body cope with the effects of alcohol, nicotine, and other pollutants. Citrus fruits, strawberries, potatoes, cabbage, tomatoes, watermelons, and green vegetables like peppers, parsley, and broccoli are all rich in vitamin C.

Does vitamin C cure the common cold? Despite the noisy controversy in the press, there is no definitive answer to that question. However, C is a natural antihistamine, which will control the running eyes and noses you get from colds and allergies.

D is for Daylight

Vitamin D helps your body absorb calcium. Since sunlight converts the chemical melanin in your skin to vitamin D, some of this vitamin comes to you naturally. Other sources of vitamin D are milk, eggs, salmon, tuna, and fish liver oil. It is rare for people who spend time outdoors and drink enriched milk to suffer from vitamin D deficiency.

E is for Energy

Muscle tone and the storage of glycogen are improved by vitamin E. This vitamin is plentiful in whole wheat, wheat germ, peanuts, fresh almonds, and sunflower seeds. Whole wheat bread contains seven times the amount of vitamin E found in white bread.

In recent years, many physicians have been prescribing vitamin E for breast cysts. This vitamin, when applied directly to affected skin, also has been found to promote healing of scarred skin, chapped lips, and sores.

Many vitamins found in fresh foods are depleted by overcooking and exposure to light. So for the sake of your vitamins, balance your diet with fresh foods. If you decide to take a vitamin supplement, avoid brands that contain sugar, starch, salt preservatives, and artificial coloring.

Be kind to yourself. Take the time to get out of the smog and into a nice warm relaxing bath. Cut down on coffee and fast foods and treat yourself to a healthy diet of fresh foods. Set aside time to exercise and be proud of the stronger, healthier you.

● ●

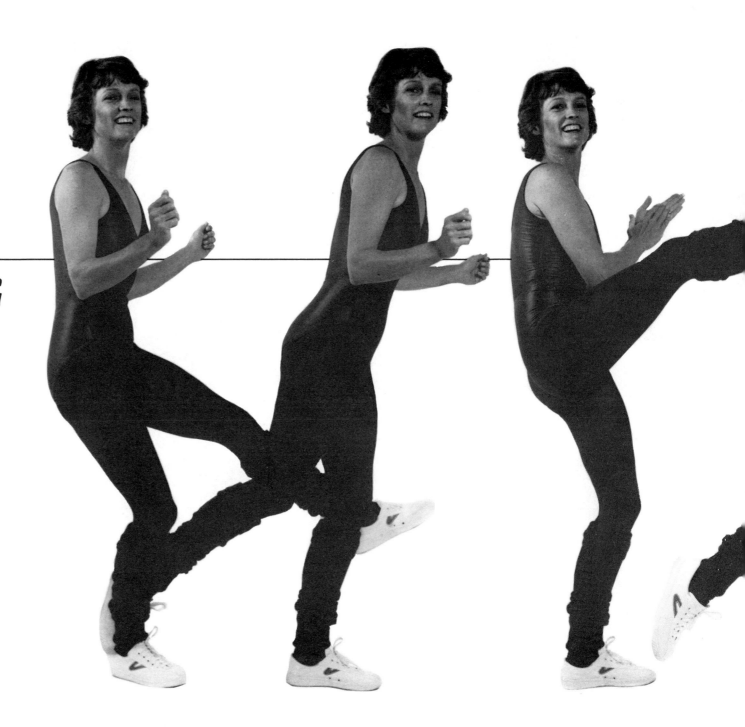

STICKING
WITH IT

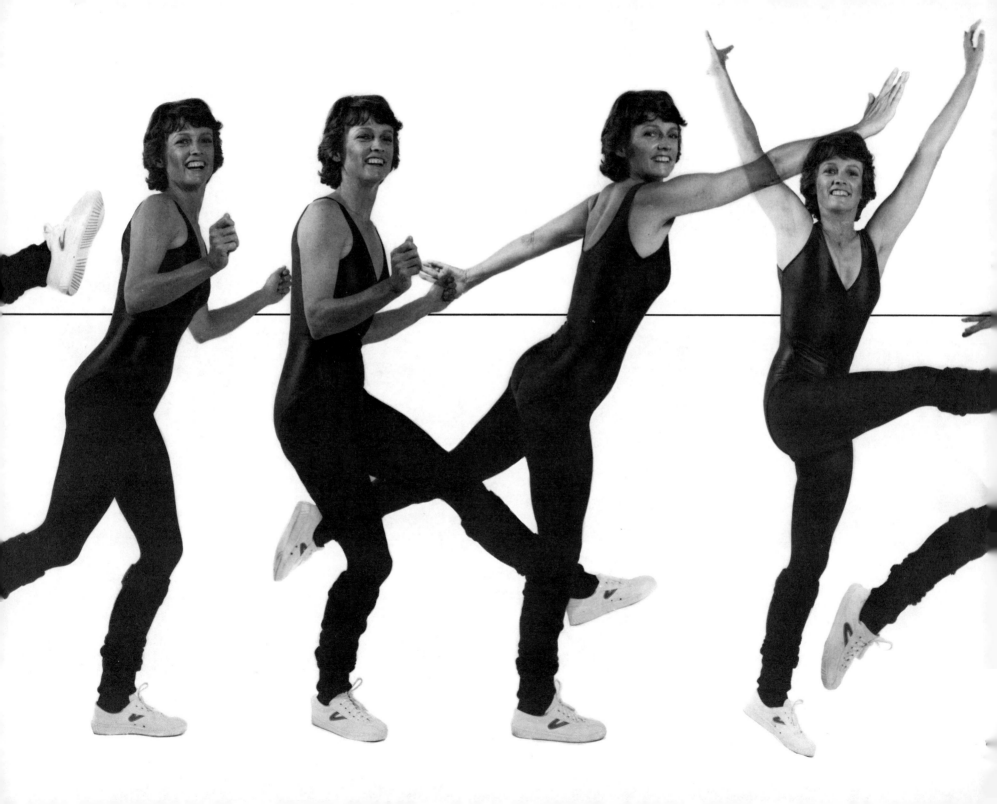

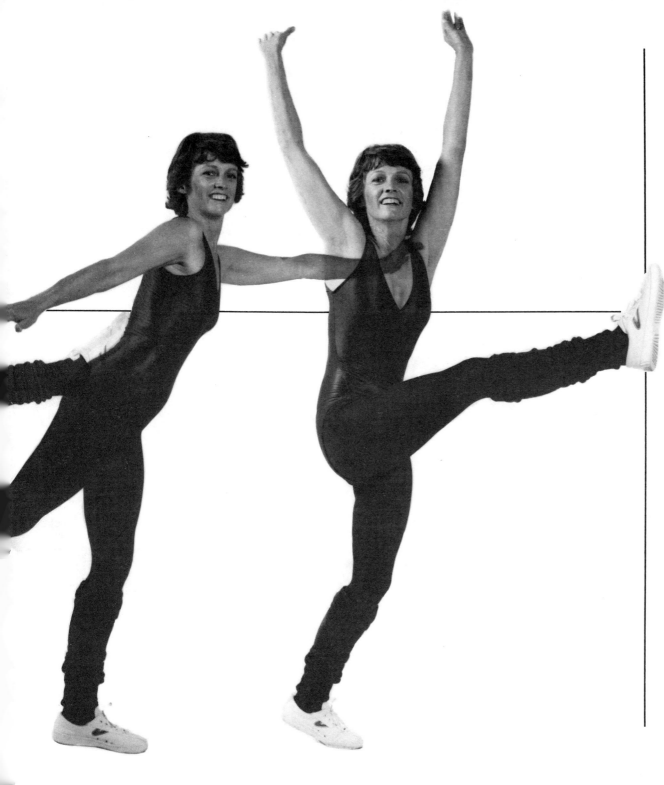

Personalizing Aerobic Slimnastics

Now you know the Aerobic Slimnastics exercises. If you have worked through all the advanced exercises, you have 18 routines and over 150 exercises in your repertoire and can design a personal program by mixing and matching them. Follow the basic Aerobic Slimnastics format:

1. Slow standing warm-up.

2. Walking warm-up.

3. Kick routine at a chair.

4. Pelvic shifts and/or a disco routine.

5. Aerobic routines—use a variety of exercises from Aerobic Highs I, II, and III.

Be sure you take and record your pulse. Have your drink of water.
Move right into:

6. Standing slimnastics.

7. Slimnastic routines for hips and thighs, buttocks, legs, and abdominals, concentrating on your problem areas.

8. Sit-ups at the level that's correct for you.

9. Slow seated cool-down stretch.

10. Sexercise.

Finish up with your drink of water.

Before each workout, plan your program carefully. Stick to your plan, but be sure to evaluate each session afterwards, noting which exercises were particularly challenging. Vary the body of the program as you like, but always include the warm-up and the sexercises. Be sure you exercise the total body from head to toe.

Continue to record your progress. Note your active pulse rate after peak and your cool-down pulse rate after sexercise. Pay attention to the parts of your body that feel good, those that feel stiff, and those that need more work. Read your emotional thermometer—what are the movements that made you feel joyful and alive and left you looking forward to your next Aerobic Slimnastics session.

•••••••••••••••••••••••••••••••••••

Evaluating Exercise Programs

Share the joy of fitness with others. Join us in an Aerobic Slimnastics class. If there is not one nearby, you can evaluate other exercise programs in your area with your newly gained expertise and a few tips. There are many programs available today, so you have the opportunity to be a conscientious consumer.

Your instructor should be a fitness missionary who believes physical fitness can change your life not only physically, but emotionally and spiritually too. Look for a person who truly enjoys teaching, has a sense of humor, and is enthusias-

tic enough to make the class fun for everyone. An effective teacher should face the class, be on the lookout for struggling students, and be able to correct difficulties with the exercises. The instructor should pay careful attention to back safety, pelvic and knee work, shin splints, cramps, stitches, and aerobic conditioning.

Look for a careful warm-up, a comfortable blend of aerobics and slimnastics, and an ade-

quate cool-down. The pace of the class should be challenging, but students ought to be encouraged to work at their own level. Routines should be easy to follow. If the footwork is too complicated, you will find yourself struggling with two left feet, and this will so encumber you that you will be unable to reach your goals of aerobic conditioning. The class atmosphere should be friendly, supportive, and fun.

•••

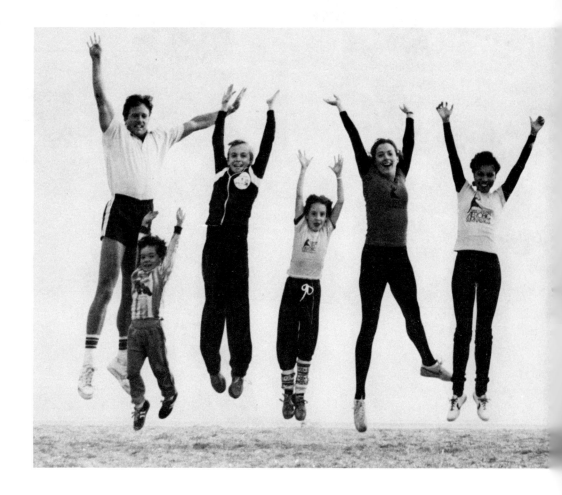

Celebrating

We're fitness friends. We've exercised together through Aerobic Slimnastics. I hope I've inspired you to enjoy exercise as I do. I know you've found new energy, self-confidence, and strength. We've worked together, but you've done it for yourself. Give yourself a pat on the back and a big hug. Have a drink of water on me. It's time to *celebrate*.

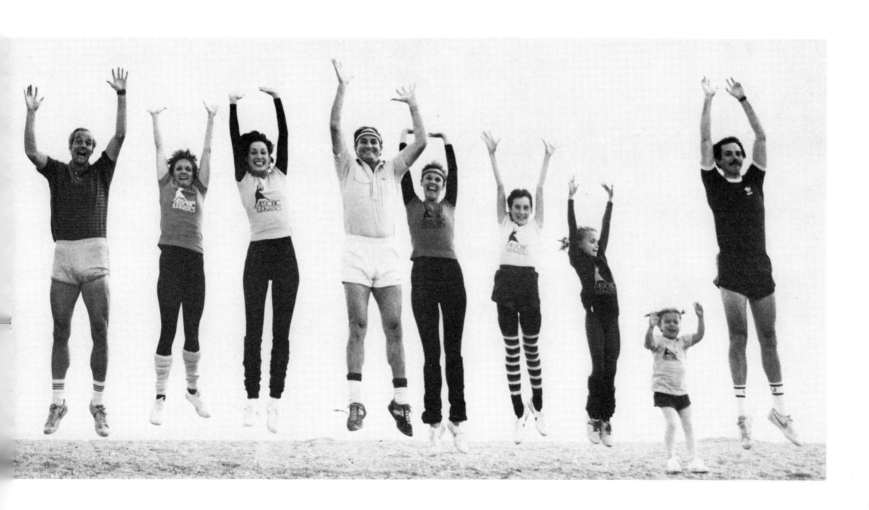

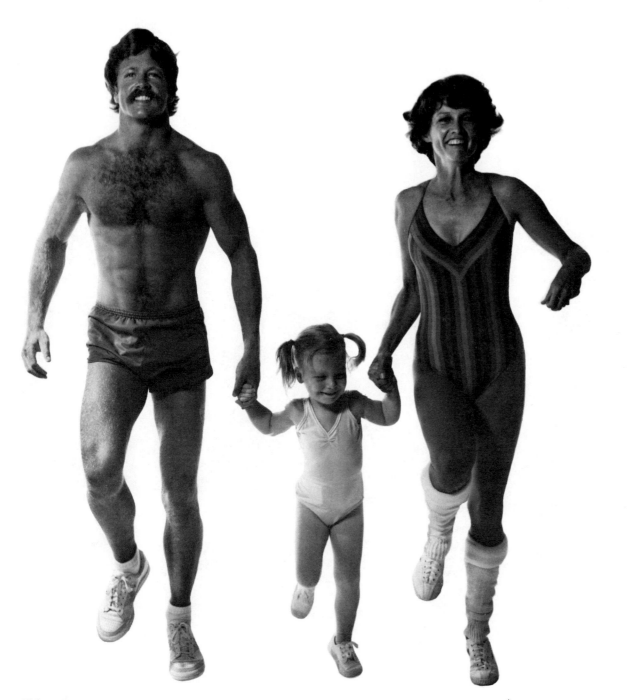

References and Recommended Reading

BOOKS

Brody, Jane. *Jane Brody's Nutrition Book.* New York: Norton, 1981.

Cooking Without Your Salt Shaker. American Heart Association. Northeast Ohio Affiliate in Cooperation with Cleveland Dietetic Association, 1978.

Cooper, Kenneth, M.D., M.P.H. *Aerobics.* New York: Bantam Books, 1968.

Deutsch, Ronald M. *Key to Feminine Response in Marriage.* New York: Random House, 1968.

———. *Realities of Nutrition.* Palo Alto, California: Bull Publishing Company, 1976.

Gilmore, C.P., and editors of Time-Life Books. *Exercising for Fitness.* Alexandria, Virginia: Time-Life Books, 1981.

Goulart, Frances Sheridan. *Eating to Win.* New York: Day Books, Stein and Day, 1982.

Mirkin, Gabe, M.D., and Hoffman, Marshall. *The Sportsmedicine Book.* Boston/Toronto: Little Brown and Co., 1978.

Noble, Elizabeth. *Essential Exercises for the Childbearing Years.* Boston: Houghton Mifflin, 1982.

Nyad, Diana, and Hogan, Candace Lyle. *Diana Nyad's Basic Training for Women.* New York: Harmony Books, 1981.

Prudden, Bonnie. *How to Keep Slender and Fit After Thirty.* New York: Pocket Books, 1969.

Shapiro, Howard I., M.D. *The Birth Control Book,* New York: Avon, 1978.

ARTICLES

Avena, Sherry. "How to Have a Healthy Heart." *Shape,* February 1982, pp. 28–32.

Bennett, William, and Gurin, Joel. "Do Diets Really Work?" *Science '82,* March 1982, pp. 42–50.

Gottlieb, William. "Vitamin Directory." *Women's Sports,* December 1980, pp. 27–42.

"More Than a Drop to Drink." *Women's Sports,* August 1981, pp. 52.

Hartbarger, Janie and Neil. "Carbohydrates." *Runner's World,* March 1982, pp. 32–35.

Hoover, Sue. "The Fats of Life: A Look at Body Composition Testing." *Women's Sports,* October 1980, pp. 18–20.

"Encyclopedia of Minerals." *Women's Sports,* March 1981, pp. 40–45.

Pearce, Richard, Ph.D. "Body Fluids." *Runner's World,* April 1982, pp. 45–48.

"Salt: A New Villain?" *Time,* March 15, 1982, pp. 64–71.

Shuer, Marjorie. "Steroids." *Women's Sports,* April 1982, pp. 17–23.

PAMPHLETS

Staid, Kay. *Nutrition and You.* Westport, Connecticut: 1981. Write c/o Aerobic Slimnastics, 15 Oak Ridge Park, Westport, Ct. 06880.

U.S. Department of Agriculture. *Nutrition and Your Health. Dietary Guidelines for Americans: 1981.* Write to U.S. Department of Agriculture, Center for Science in the Public Interest, 1755 S. Street, N.W., Washington, D.C. 20009. (Bulk prices available.) 1981. 18 pgs.

CHARTS

Jacobson, Michael, Ph.D. "Chemical Cuisine." U.S. Department of Agriculture, Center for Science in the Public Interest, 1775 S. Street, N.W., Washington, DC, 20009.

Zimmerman, Jean. "Nutrition Scoreboard." U.S. Department of Agriculture, Center for Science in the Public Interest, 1775 S. Street, N.W., Washington, DC, 20009.

•••••••••••••••••••••••••••••••••••••

Index

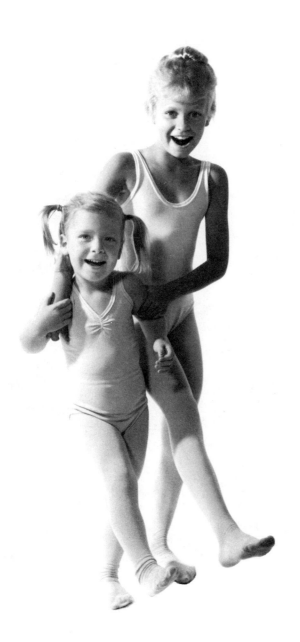

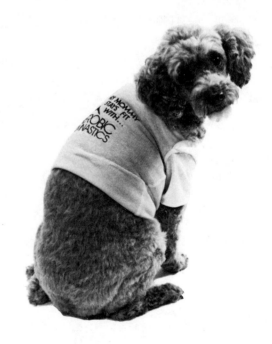